# SIMPLE QIGONG EXERCISES FOR HEALTH

# Simple Qigong Exercises for Health

## Improve Your Health in 10 to 20 Minutes a Day
## The Eight Pieces of Brocade

健身八段錦

### By
### Dr. Yang, Jwing-Ming

YMAA Publication Center, Inc.
Wolfeboro NH USA

**YMAA Publication Center, Inc.**
PO Box 480
Wolfeboro, NH 03894
800 669-8892 • www.ymaa.com • info@ymaa.com

Paperback ISBN: 9781594392696
Ebook ISBN: 9781594392672
Enhanced Ebook ISBN: 9781594392658

Cover design by Axie Breen
Copyedit by Dolores Sparrow
Proofreading by Sara Scanlon
Editorial supervision by Susan Bullowa

Photos by YMAA unless noted otherwise.

POD 1115

### Publisher's Cataloging in Publication

Yang, Jwing-Ming, 1946-

Simple qigong exercises for health : improve your health in 10 to 20 minutes a day : the eight pieces of brocade / by Yang, Jwing-Ming. -- Wolfeboro, NH : YMAA Publication Center, c2013.

p. ; cm.

ISBN: 978-1-59439-269-6 (pbk) ; 978-1-59439-267-2 (ebook)
Revision of "Eight simple qigong exercises for health" (2nd ed., YMAA Publication Center, 1997).
Includes bibliographical references and index.
Summary: The book offers beginners a smart way to learn qigong, the ancient Chinese system of gentle breathing, stretching, and strengthening movements. Using 'The Eight Pieces of Brocade', one of the most popular qigong healing exercise sets, students can choose the sitting set, the standing set, or both, to improve overall health and well-being.--Publisher.

1. Qi gong. 2. Qi (Chinese philosphy) 3. Medicine, Chinese. 4. Mind and body. 5. Holistic medicine. I. Title. II. Title: Eight simple qigong exercises for health.

RA781.8 .Y3633 2013          2013949311

613.7/1489--dc23          1310

The practice, treatments, and methods described in this book should not be used as an alternative to professional medical diagnosis or treatment. The authors and publisher of this book are NOT RESPONSIBLE in any manner whatsoever for any injury or negative effects, which may occur through following the instructions and advise, contained herein.

It is recommended that before beginning any treatment or exercise program, you consult your medical professional to determine whether you should undertake this course of practice.

Printed in USA.

# Romanization of Chinese Words

The interior of this book primarily uses the Pinyin Romanization system of Chinese to English. In some instances, a more popular word may be used as an aid for reader convenience, such as 'tai chi' in place of the Pinyin spelling taiji. Pinyin is standard in the People's Republic of China and in several world organizations, including the United Nations. Pinyin, which was introduced in China in the 1950s, replaces the older Wade-Giles and Yale systems.

Some common conversions are found in the following:

| Pinyin | Also Spelled as | Pronunciation |
|--------|-----------------|---------------|
| qi | chi | chē |
| qigong | chi Kung | chē gōng |
| qin na | chin Na | chǐn nǎ |
| jin | jing | jǐn |
| gongfu | kung fu | gōng foo |
| taijiquan | tai chi chuan | tī jē chǔén |

For more information, please refer to *The People's Republic of China: Administrative Atlas, The Reform of the Chinese Written Language*, or a contemporary manual of style.

# Formats and Treatment for Chinese Words

The first instances of foreign words are set in italics.

Transliterations are provided frequently. For example: Eight Pieces of Brocade (Ba Duan Jin, 八段錦).

Chinese persons' names are mostly presented in their more popular spelling (Romanization). Capitalization is according to the Chicago Manual of Style 16th edition. The author or publisher may use a specific spelling or capitalization use as respect to the living or deceased person. For example: Cheng, Man-ch'ing vs. Zheng Manqing.

Chapters 3 and 4. Chinese poetry is followed by the author's translation with commentary.

# Contents

# Preface First Edition (1988)

Since my first qigong book, *Chi Kung—Health and Martial Arts,* was published, I have received countless letters and phone calls. Almost all of them are to express people's gratitude for the benefit they have received from practicing the qigong exercises introduced in the book. Surprisingly, many of the readers are Western doctors who have been applying qigong theory and teaching the exercises to their patients and obtaining very positive results. Many of them have suggested that I produce videotapes to help people learn the exercises more accurately and efficiently.

With this encouragement, I have been studying and researching more deeply, trying to increase my understanding of the exercises. After three years of study and practice, I have decided to publish the following videotapes. The first tape will introduce one of the most common and basic qigong exercises in China—The Eight Pieces of Brocade (*Ba Duan Jin*, 八段錦). This set of exercises was created by Marshal Yue, Fei (岳飛) during the Southern Song dynasty (南宋) (AD 1127–1279) for improving his soldiers' health. Since that time, these exercises have become one of the most popular sets in China.

There are a number of reasons for introducing this set first:

1. Its theory and training methods are the simplest and easiest to understand. It is therefore the best set for the qigong beginner.
2. If you practice this set regularly, you should notice improvements in your health within a few months.
3. The set can be practiced by anyone, young or old, healthy or sick.
4. This set will give you a good understanding of basic qigong theory so that if you wish, you may go on to more advanced training.

Although it is best to use this manual together with the videotape, it is possible to learn the set using this manual alone. Seeing the set done will clear up many small questions and avoid the ambiguities inherent in any printed description or still photograph. However, if you read carefully and proceed step by step, you should be able to grasp the essentials well enough to gain full benefit from the exercises.

If there proves to be enough of a demand for manuals and videotapes such as these, YMAA will publish a continuing series of qigong training materials. These materials will introduce a number of different qigong sets and explain the theoretical background for each. At present, a series of ten videotapes and manuals is envisioned, ranging from basic to advanced.

In addition, I am working on a series of books that will discuss in greater depth the various styles of qigong. The first book will lay down the theoretical foundation, or root, of qigong. This book will give you a general understanding of the theory and principles, which is necessary if you wish to further your study. The second book in this series will be on Muscle/Tendon Changing and Marrow/Brain Washing Qigong (易筋經，洗髓經). This qigong has been known in China (although it has been kept secret) since the Liang dynasty (梁), more than fourteen hundred years ago. Muscle/Tendon Changing and Marrow/Brain Washing is deep and difficult to understand, but once mastered it can give you the health of a child, increase your resistance to disease, and even lengthen your life.

The third volume will be concerned with Qigong Cavity Press Healing. It will help people understand the basic principles of acupressure. Qigong Cavity Press Healing is the root of Japanese Shiatsu Massage. The fourth volume will cover qigong and health, including basic principles as well as various styles of qigong designed to improve health or to treat specific ailments. The next volume will concern qigong training that the martial artist can use to improve his fighting potential, such as Shaolin Qigong training methods, iron shirt, and iron sand palm. Further volumes will introduce Tibetan, Daoist, and Buddhist (*Chan* or *Ren*, 禪 or 忍) meditation methods.

As you can see, this is a very ambitious undertaking, and I can foresee a number of difficulties both in finance and in writing. It will be a new challenge for YMAA and me, and it will take many years of effort to complete. However, with your support and encouragement, we will complete it, even if it takes longer than anticipated.

This manual will start by briefly introducing in the first two chapters the history of qigong and the fundamental theory. The third and fourth chapters in this volume will introduce the sitting and the standing sets of the Eight Pieces of Brocade.

Practicing qigong (which is working with qi, the energy within the body) cannot only maintain your health and mental balance, but can also cure a number of illnesses without the use of any drugs. Qigong uses either still or moving meditation to increase and regulate the qi circulation.

When you practice regularly, your mind will gradually become calm and peaceful, and your whole being will start to feel more balanced. However, the most important thing that will come from the regular practice of qigong is your discovery of the inner world of your body's energy. Through sensing and feeling, and examining your inner experiences, you will start to understand yourself not only physically but also mentally. This science of internal sensing, which the Chinese have been studying for several thousand years, is usually totally ignored by the Western world. However, in today's busy and confusing society, this training is especially important. With the mental peace and calmness that qigong can give you, you will be better able to relax and enjoy your daily work and perhaps even find real happiness.

I believe that it is very important for the Western world to learn, study, research, and develop this scientific internal art immediately, and on a wide scale. I sincerely believe that it can be very effective in helping people, especially young people, to cope with the confusing and frightening challenges of life. The general practice of qigong could reduce the mental pressure in our society, help those who are unbalanced, and perhaps even lower the crime rate. Qigong balances the internal energy and can heal many illnesses. Older people especially will find that it will maintain their health and even slow the aging process. In addition, qigong will help older people conquer depression and worry, and find peace, calm, and real happiness. I am confident that people in the Western world will realize, as have millions of Chinese, that qigong practice will give them a new outlook on life and that it will turn out to be a key to solving many of today's problems.

For these reasons, I have been actively studying, researching, and publishing what I have learned. However, after a few years of effort, I feel that what I have accomplished is too slow and shallow. I and the few people like me, who are struggling to spread the word about qigong, cannot do it well enough by ourselves. We need to get more people involved, but we especially need to have universities and established medical organizations get involved in the research.

To conclude, I would like to point out one thing to those of you who are sincerely interested in studying and researching this new science. If you start now, future generations will view you as a pioneer of the scientific investigation of qigong. In addition to improving your own health, you will share the credit for raising our understanding of life as well as increasing the store of happiness in this world.

# Preface Second Edition (1997)

This book, *Simple Qigong Exercises for Health* (formerly titled *The Eight Pieces of Brocade*), introduces healing qigong exercises that are more than one thousand years old. These exercises were created by Marshal Yue, Fei (岳飛) during the Chinese Southern Song dynasty. Since then, these exercises have been commonly used by the Chinese general public for health and healing. Though the exercises are very simple and easy to learn, the theory of healing is very profound, scientific, and complete. Every movement was created by imitating the natural instinctive reactions and movements that people make when they feel discomfort or pain (a signal from the body to notify your brain that the qi is losing balance). An example is lifting your right arm to release the stress or pressure on your liver due to fatigue or poor quality food. Another example is bowing at the waist to use the back muscles to massage and improve the circulation in the kidneys. Normally, if you do not react to these urgent calls, a physical defect or damage may occur.

Since its creation, countless healing qigong exercises were developed following the basic theory of the Eight Pieces of Brocade (*Ba Duan Jin*, 八段錦). It is called "brocade" because brocade is a shining and beautiful cloth. When you practice these exercises regularly and correctly, it is just as if you have added a shining and beautiful life force to your body.

The concept of qigong is still new in the West. In fact, this more than four-thousand-year-old healing knowledge was not introduced to the West until 1973, when President Nixon visited China and opened its long-closed door. Since then, Chinese culture has been widely imported by the West. Chinese medical science, including acupuncture, qigong exercises, and herbal treatments (which have been experienced for many thousands of years), has also seriously influenced Western society.

Since I arrived in America in 1974, I have witnessed the great cultural exchange between the East and West. I have always believed that in order to have a peaceful and harmonious world, all humans must communicate with each other so they can understand and respect each other. In order to expedite this exchange, I quit my engineering job and put all my effort into translating, teaching, and publishing ancient Chinese documents. Yang's Martial Arts Association (YMAA) was founded in 1982 and with it, I began to fulfill my dreams. YMAA Publication Center was established in 1984 and since then it has published books and videos about Chinese qigong and Chinese martial arts.

I believe that the beginning of a cultural exchange is most important. If this transition is correct, the ideas and concepts introduced will be accurate. Otherwise, the information passed on will be distorted. Once it is distorted, it is very difficult to correct the wrong path. For example, many Chinese martial arts were originally created in Buddhist and Daoist monasteries for self-discipline and moral cultivation. When these arts were introduced to the West, violent and exciting physical fighting and flashy techniques were emphasized. The inner virtues of self-challenge and spiritual cultivation were completely ignored. Naturally, this was caused by importing these arts in the wrong way—through violent Chinese martial arts fighting movies.

In recent decades, I have also seen many of China's non-medical qigong masters demonstrate mysterious and superstitious qigong power and claim this to be the right qigong. This demonstrates to me how important it is to publish more books and videos so as to introduce the correct Chinese healing arts to the West. Chinese qigong healing arts are derived from scientific and logical analysis and conclusions through thousands of years of healing and health maintenance experience. It is a traditional human medicine and its effectiveness has been verified through thousands of years of human history. The most unique and important part of qigong practice is not just obtaining physical health, but also mental internal health with a meditative mind. This mental element has commonly been ignored in Western health exercises.

This book is a first step toward understanding the science of Chinese qigong. If you are interested, you should read more documents and publications. Then use your logical mind to analyze the truth behind the practice. Only then will you have the correct feeling of the art and believe its effectiveness from your deep heart.

Since this book was first published in 1988, I have written many other qigong books, which may offer you more information. These books are the following:

**Beginner Level**

*Qigong for Health and Martial Arts—Exercises and Meditation*
*Arthritis Relief—Chinese Qigong for Healing & Prevention* (special qigong treatment)
*Back Pain Relief—Simple Qigong Exercises for Healing & Prevention* (special qigong treatment)

**Intermediate Level**

*Qigong Massage—Fundamental Techniques for Health and Relaxation*

**Advanced Level**

*The Root of Chinese Qigong—Secrets for Health, Longevity, and Enlightenment*
*Qigong, The Secret of Youth—Da Mo's Muscle Tendon and Marrow Brain Washing Qigong Classics*
*The Essence of Shaolin White Crane—Martial Power and Qigong*

Companion videos are also available for many of the above publications from YMAA Publication Center.

The new edition of this book has been updated from the old edition in several ways. First, the Chinese Romanization system has been changed to Pinyin, which has become more popular and widely accepted by Western academic scholars. Second, many Chinese characters have been included in the text for those who can read Chinese. Third, a glossary has been added for better reference. Fourth, many new photos have been added. Finally, an index has also been provided for your convenience.

Dr. Yang, Jwing-Ming
President, YMAA International
January 28, 1997

# Acknowledgments

### First Edition (1988)

Thanks to A. Reza Farman-Farmaian for the photography, to David Ripianzi, Dave Sollars, Eric Hoffman, and James O'Leary, Jr. for proofing the manuscript and for contributing many valuable suggestions and discussions, and to Christer Manning for the drawings and cover design. Special thanks to Alan Dougall for his editing.

### Second Edition (1997)

In this new edition, I would like to express many thanks to Tim Comrie for typesetting and photography, to Kathy K. Yang, Nicholas C. Yang, and Mei-Ling Yang for general help, to Kain M. Sanderson and Jeff Grace for proofing, and to Andrew Murray for his editing. Thanks also to Ilana Rosenberg for her cover design.

### Second Edition Revision (2013)

The publisher wishes to thank Axie Breen for the cover design, Dolores Sparrow for copyediting, Sara Scanlon for proofreading, and Susan Bullowa for digital file management.

# Chapter 1. General Introduction

## 1-1. Introduction

If you study the history of the human race, you will see that a large part of this history has been taken up with war, conquest, killing, and the struggle for power. We have tended to worship as heroes those who could conquer and rule other countries, and we have wrongly educated each new generation to glorify killing and slavery, and to worship power. There have been only relatively short periods when humankind has not been at war, when people could live their lives in peace and tranquility; but it was during these times that people created art, wrote poems, and sought ways to live longer and happier lives.

In their seven thousand years of history, the Chinese people have experienced all possible human suffering and pain. Chinese culture is like a seven-thousand-year-old man who has seen and experienced all of the pain of human life. Yet through his experience, he has also accumulated a great store of knowledge. China's long spiritual experience cannot be compared to the popular culture of the West, which is the result of centuries of emphasis on the material sciences, money, war, and conquest. If you research Chinese culture through its literature and painting, you will discover that they rank among the greatest achievements of the human spirit. They reflect humankind's joy and grief, pleasure and suffering, peace and strife, vitality, sickness, and death.

Coming from this complex cultural and historical background, the Chinese people have long sought ways of living healthy and happy lives. However, while on the one hand the Chinese study themselves spiritually, they also tend to say that everything that happens is destiny and is prearranged by heaven. While holding the fatalistic belief that everything is predetermined, the Chinese also looked for ways to resist the apparent inevitability of sickness and death.

It was with this seemingly contradictory and no-win point of view that the Chinese focused their attention on self-study and self-cultivation. This inward feeling and looking, this spiritual searching, has become one of the major roots of Chinese culture and medical science. Once *qi*, or the internal energy within the human body, was discovered, it was studied very carefully. When the link between the qi in the human body and the qi in nature was discovered, the hope soon grew that this qi was the means whereby humans could escape from the trap of sickness and death. When viewed from this historical background, it is not difficult to understand why a major part of Chinese culture, other than warfare, was based on the religions of Daoism and Buddhism, and spiritual science.

So many people today are devoting all their efforts striving for, and even achieving, material wealth, and yet they are suffering spiritually. They wander through their lives, listlessly or frantically, wondering what it is they are missing. Their lives have no meaning or purpose. Many seek temporary release from their pain through drugs. I deeply believe that if these people were to study the spiritual practices that have been developed over these several thousand years, they would find the mental balance, which is especially necessary for today's society.

In this chapter, we will first define qi and *qigong*, and then survey the history of qigong. This will be followed by the story of the creator of the Eight Pieces of Brocade. Finally, qigong theory and training principles will be discussed.

## 1-2. Definition of Qi and Qigong

### What is Qi?

In order to understand qigong, you must first understand qi. Qi is the energy or natural force that fills the universe. There are three general types of qi. Heaven (the sky or universe) has heaven qi (*tian qi*, 天氣), which is made up of the forces that the heavenly bodies exert on the earth, such as sunshine, moonlight, and the moon's effect on the tides. The earth has earth qi (*di qi*, 地氣), which absorbs the heaven qi and is influenced by it. Humans have human qi (*ren qi*, 人氣), which is influenced by the other two. In ancient times, the Chinese believed that it was heaven qi that controlled the weather, climate, and natural disasters. When this qi or energy field loses its balance, it strives to rebalance itself. Then the wind must blow, rain must fall, and even tornadoes and hurricanes must happen in order for the heaven qi to reach a new energy balance. Heaven qi also affects human qi, and divination and astrology are attempts to explain this.

Under heaven qi is earth qi. It is influenced and controlled by heaven qi. For example, too much rain will force a river to flood or change its path. Without rain, the plants will die. The Chinese believe that earth qi is made up of lines and patterns of energy, as well as the earth's magnetic field and the heat concealed underground. These energies must also balance; otherwise, disasters such as earthquakes will occur. When the qi of the earth is balanced, plants will grow and animals will prosper. Also, each individual person, animal, and plant has its own qi field, which always seeks to be balanced. When any individual living thing loses its balance, it will sicken, die, and decompose.

You must understand that all natural things, including humans, grow within and are influenced by the natural cycles of heaven qi and earth qi. Since you are part of this nature (*Dao*, 道), you must understand heaven qi and earth qi. Then you will be able to adjust yourself, when necessary, to fit more smoothly into the natural cycle, and you will learn how to protect yourself from the negative influences in nature. This is the major goal of qigong practice.

From this, you can see that in order to have a long and healthy life, the first rule is that you must live in harmony with the cycles of nature and avoid and prevent the negative influences. The Chinese have researched nature for thousands of years. Some of the information on the patterns and cycles of nature has been recorded in books, one of which is the *Book of Changes* (*Yi Jing*, 易經). This book gives the average person formulas to trace when the season will change, when it will snow, when a farmer should plow or harvest. You must remember that nature is always repeating itself. If you observe carefully, you will be able to see many of these routine patterns and cycles caused by the rebalancing of the qi fields.

Over thousands of years, the Chinese have researched the interrelationships of all things in nature, especially about human beings. From this experience, they have created various qigong exercises to help bring the body's qi circulation into harmony with nature's cycles. This helps to avoid illnesses caused by weather or seasonal changes.

After a long period of research and study, the Chinese also discovered that through qigong practice they were able to strengthen their qi or internal energy circulation, and slow down the degeneration of the body, gaining not only health but also a longer life. The realization that such things were possible greatly spurred new research.

## What is Qigong?

From the above discussion, you can see that qi is energy and is found in heaven, in the earth, and in every living thing. All of these different types of energy interact with each other and can convert into each other. In China, the word "*gong*" (功) is often used instead of "*gongfu*" (功夫), which means energy and time. Any study or training that requires a lot of energy and time to learn or to accomplish is called gongfu. The term can be applied to any special skill or study as long as it requires time, energy, and patience. Therefore, the correct definition of qigong is any training or study dealing with qi that takes a long time and a lot of effort.

Qi exists in everything. Since the range of qi is so vast, the Chinese have divided it into three categories, parallel to the three natural powers (*san cai*, 三才) of heaven, earth, and man. Generally speaking, heaven qi is the biggest and the most powerful. This heaven qi contains within it the earth qi, and within this heaven and earth qi lives humans, with their own qi. You can see from the diagram that human qi is part of heaven and earth qi. However, since the human beings who research qi are mainly interested in human qi, the term qigong is generally used to refer only to qi training for people.

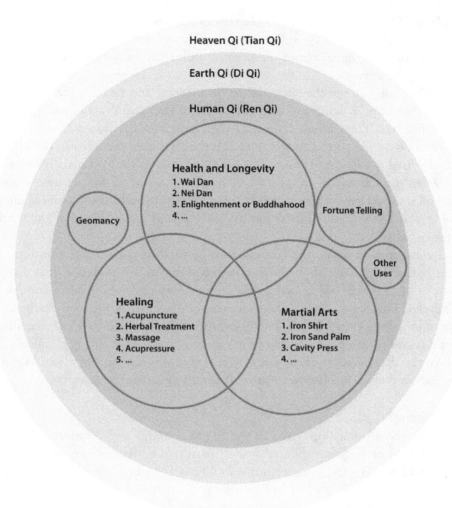

Heaven Qi (Tian Qi)

Earth Qi (Di Qi)

Human Qi (Ren Qi)

**Health and Longevity**
1. Wai Dan
2. Nei Dan
3. Enlightenment or Buddhahood
4. ...

Geomancy

Fortune Telling

Other Uses

**Healing**
1. Acupuncture
2. Herbal Treatment
3. Massage
4. Acupressure
5. ...

**Martial Arts**
1. Iron Shirt
2. Iron Sand Palm
3. Cavity Press
4. ...

Qi diagram.

As you can see, qigong research should include heaven qi, earth qi, and human qi. Understanding heaven qi is very difficult, however, and it was especially so in ancient times when the science was just developing. The major rules and principles relating to heaven qi can be found in such books as *The Five Elements and Ten Stems* (*Wuxing and Shitiangan*, 五行與十天干); *Celestial Stems* (*Shierdizhi*, 十二地支); and the *Yi Jing* (易經).

Many people have become proficient in the study of earth qi. They are called geomancy teachers (*di li shi*, 地理師) or wind water teachers (*feng shui shi*, 風水師). These experts use the accumulated body of geomantic knowledge and the *Yi Jing* to help people make important decisions, such as where and how to build a house or even where to locate a grave. This profession is still quite common in China.

The Chinese people believe that human qi is affected and controlled by heaven qi and earth qi and that they in fact determine your destiny. Some people specialize in explaining these connections; they are called calculate life teachers (*suan ming shi*, 算命師) or fortune tellers.

Most qigong research has focused on human qi. Since qi is the source of life, if you understand how qi functions and know how to affect it correctly, you should be able to live a long and healthy life. Many different aspects of human qi have been researched, including acupuncture, acupressure, herbal treatment, meditation, and qigong exercises. The use of acupuncture, acupressure, and herbal treatment to adjust human qi flow has become the root of Chinese medical science. Meditation and moving qigong exercises are widely used by the Chinese people to improve their health or even to cure certain illnesses. Meditation and qigong exercises serve an additional role in that Daoists and Buddhists use them in their spiritual pursuit of enlightenment and Buddhahood.

You can see that the study of any of the aspects of qi should be called qigong. However, since the term is ordinarily used today only in reference to the cultivation of human qi, we will use it only in this narrower sense to avoid confusion.

## 1-3. The History of Qigong

Chinese qigong history can be divided roughly into three periods. The history of the first period is vague, although it is considered to have started when the *Book of Changes* (*Yi Jing*, 易經) was introduced to the Chinese people sometime before 2400 BC and to extend until the Han dynasty (漢) (206 BC) when Buddhism and its meditation methods were imported from India. This led qigong practice and meditation into the second period, the religious qigong era. This period lasted until the Liang dynasty (梁) (AD 502–557), when it was discovered that qigong could be used for martial purposes, which started the third period, martial qigong. In this third period, different martial qigong styles were created based on theories and principles from Buddhist and Daoist qigong. This period lasted until the overthrow of the Qing dynasty in 1911 when a new era started in which Chinese qigong training was being mixed with qigong practices from India, Japan, and many other countries.

### Before the Han Dynasty, 206 BC

When the *Book of Changes* (*Yi Jing*, 2400 BC) was introduced to the Chinese people, they believed that natural energy or power included heaven (*tian*, 天), earth (*di*, 地), and human (*ren*, 人). These were called the three natural powers (san cai, 三才). These three facets of nature have their definite rules and cycles. The rules never change, and the cycles repeat periodically. Therefore, if you could understand the rules and the cycles of heavenly timing (*tian shi*, 天時), you would be able to understand natural changes, such as the seasons, climate, weather, rain, snow, drought, and all other natural occurrences. Among the natural cycles are those of the day, the month, and the year, as well as cycles of twelve years and sixty years.

If you understand the rules and the structure of the earth, you will be able to understand geography, how plants grow, how rivers move, where is the best place to live, where to build a house and which direction it should face so that it is a healthy place to live, and many other things related to the earth. As mentioned earlier, in China today there are people who make their living in the profession called geomancy (*di li*, 地理) or wind water (*feng shui*, 風水). Feng shui is commonly used because the location and character of the wind and water in a landscape are the most important factors in evaluating a location. Feng shui professionals help people choose where to live, where to bury their dead, and even how to rearrange or redecorate homes and offices so that they are better places in which to live and work.

When you understand human relations (*ren shi*, 人事), you will be able to understand the relationship between nature and people, interpersonal relationships, and the destiny of an individual. If you understand the three natural powers, you will be able to predict natural disasters, the fate of a country, or the future of a person. The Chinese believe that in this universe it is the qi, or natural energy, which demonstrates these natural rules and cycles. This natural force decides everything, makes the plants grow, affects the birth of a child, and influences the destiny of a country, or even a person's desires and temperament. This field has generated a profession called calculate life (suan ming, 算命), which is devoted to fortune telling.

It is easy to understand that you were formed and grew under the influence of natural rules and cycles. You are part of nature, and you are channeled into the cycles of nature. If you go against this natural cycle, you will become sick and soon die. If you know the natural cycles and learn how to live with them, you will gain a long and healthy life. That is the meaning of "Dao," which can be translated as "the natural way."

Based on the understanding of these principles, the Chinese people figured out a way to calculate the changes of natural qi. This calculation is called the eight trigrams (*bagua*, 八卦). From the eight trigrams are derived the 64 hexagrams. Therefore, the *Yi Jing* was probably the first book that taught the Chinese people about qi and its variations in nature and man. The relationship of the three natural powers and their qi variations were later discussed extensively in the book *Theory of Qi's Variation* (*Qi Hua Lun*, 氣化論).

Around 1766–1154 BC, during the Shang dynasty (商), Chinese doctors started using stone probes called "*bian shi*" (砭石) to adjust people's qi circulation. This is considered the beginning of acupuncture. During the Zhou dynasty (周) (1122–934 BC), Lao Zi (老子), also called Li, Er (李耳), described certain breathing techniques in his

*Classic on the Virtue of the Dao* (*Dao De Jing*, 道德經). Later, *Historical Record* (*Shi Ji*, 史記) in the Spring and Autumn and Warring States Periods (春秋戰國) (770–221 BC) also described more complete methods of breath training. About 300 BC, the Daoist philosopher Zhuang Zi (莊子) described the relationship between health and breath.

During the Qin and Han dynasties, (秦，漢) (221 BC–AD 220), several books were written that discussed the circulation of qi: *The Classic on Disorders* (*Nan Jing*, 難經) by Bian Que (扁鵲); *Prescriptions from the Golden Chamber* (*Jin*

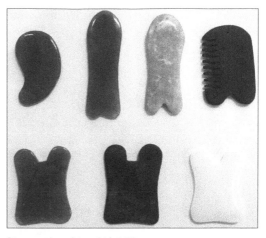

Stone probes, bian shi (砭石).

*Kui Yao Lue*, 金匱要略) by Zhang, Zhong-jing (張仲景); and *A Comparative Study of the Jou (dynasty) Book of Changes* (*Zhou Yi Can Tong Qi*, 周易參同契) by Wei, Bo-yang (魏伯陽). It can be seen from this list that up to this time, almost all of the publications were written by scholars such as Lao Zi and Zhuang Zi, or medical doctors such as Bian Que and Wei, Bo-yang. Characteristics of qigong in this period were as follows:

1. There were two major types of qigong training. One type was used by the Confucian (*Rujia*, 儒家) and Daoist (*Daojia*, 道家) scholars, who used it primarily to maintain their health. The other type of qigong was for medical purposes, using needles or exercises to adjust the qi or to cure illness.

2. Except for Daoism, there was almost no religious color to the training.

3. All of the training was passive rather than active, gently improving and maintaining health.

## After the Han Dynasty and before the Liang Dynasty, c. AD 502

In China, the Han dynasty was a glorious and peaceful period. It was during the Eastern Han dynasty (東漢) (c. AD 58) that Buddhism was imported to China from India. Because the Han emperor was a sincere Buddhist, Buddhism soon spread and became very popular. Many Buddhist meditation and qigong practices, which had been practiced in India for thousands of years, were absorbed into the Chinese culture. The Buddhist temples taught many qigong practices, especially still meditation (*Chan* or *Ren*, 禪 or 忍), which marked a new era of qigong practice. Much of the deeper qigong theory and practices that had been developed in India were brought to China. Unfortunately, since the training was directed at attaining Buddhahood, the training practices and theory were recorded in the Buddhist bibles and kept secret. For hundreds of years the religious qigong training was never taught to laymen. Only in this century has it been available to the general populace.

Not long after Buddhism was imported into China, a Daoist by the name of Zhang, Dao-ling (張道陵) combined the traditional Daoist principles with Buddhism and created a religion called *Dao Jiao* (道教). Many of the meditation methods were a combination of the principles and training methods of both sources.

Since Tibet had its own branch of Buddhism with its own training system and methods of attaining Buddhahood, Tibetan Buddhists were also invited to China to preach. In time, their practices were also absorbed.

In addition to the qigong meditations passed down secretly within the monasteries, traditional scholars and physicians continued their qigong research. During the Jin dynasty (晋) in the third century AD, a famous physician named Hua Tuo (華佗) used acupuncture for anesthesia in surgery. The Daoist Jun Qian (君倩) used the movements of animals to create the Five Animal Sports (*Wu Qin Xi*, 五禽戲), which taught people how to increase their qi circulation (some say that the Wu Qin Xi was created by Hua Tuo). Also, in this period, a physician named Ge Hong (葛洪) mentioned using the mind to lead and increase qi in his book *Embracing Simplicity* (*Bao Pu Zi*, 抱朴子). In the period AD 420–581, Tao, Hong-jing (陶弘景) compiled the *Records of Nourishing the Body and Extending Life* (*Yang Shen Yan Ming Lu*, 養身延命錄), which showed many qigong techniques. Characteristics of qigong during this period were the following:

1. There were three schools of religious qigong that influenced and dominated the qigong practice in this period. They were Indian Buddhism, Tibetan Buddhism, and Daoism.

2. Almost all of the religious qigong practices were kept secret within the monasteries.

3. Religious qigong training worked to escape from the cycle of reincarnation.

4. Relatively speaking, religious qigong theory is harder to understand than the theory of the non-religious qigong, and the training is more difficult.

5. Qi circulation theory was better understood by this time, so the qigong sets created in this period seem to be more efficient than the older sets.

### From the Liang Dynasty to the Late Qing Dynasty, c. AD 1911

During the Liang dynasty (梁) (AD 502–557), the emperor invited an Indian prince named Da Mo (達摩), who was also a Buddhist monk, to preach Buddhism in China. When the emperor decided he did not like Da Mo's Buddhist theory, the monk retreated to the Shaolin temple (少林寺). When Da Mo arrived at the Shaolin temple, he saw that the priests were weak and sick. He decided to shut himself away to ponder the problem. He stayed in seclusion for nine years. When he emerged, he wrote two classics: *Muscle/ Tendon Changing Classic (Yi Jin Jing, 易筋經)* and *Marrow/Brain Washing Classic (Xi Sui Jing, 洗髓經)*. The *Muscle/Tendon Changing Classic* taught the priests how to gain health and change their physical bodies from weak to strong. The *Marrow/Brain Washing Classic* taught the priests how to use the internal energy or qi to clean the bone marrow and strengthen the blood and immune system, as well as how to energize the brain and attain Buddhahood or enlightenment. Because the *Marrow/Brain Washing Classic* was more difficult to understand and practice, the training methods were passed down secretly to only a very few disciples in each generation.

After the priests practiced the Muscle/Tendon Changing exercises, they found that not only did they improve their health, but they also greatly increased their strength. When this training was integrated into the martial arts forms, it increased the effectiveness of their techniques. In addition to this martial qigong training, the Shaolin priests also created five animal styles of gongfu from watching the way the different animals fight. The animals imitated were the tiger, leopard, dragon, snake, and crane.

Outside of the monastery, development of qigong continued during the Sui and Tang dynasties (隋, 唐) (AD 581–907). Chao, Yun-fang (巢元方) compiled the *Thesis on Origins and Symptoms of Various Diseases (Zhu Bing Yuan Hou Lun, 諸病源候論)*, which is a veritable encyclopedia of qigong methods. He listed 260 different ways of increasing the qi flow. The *Thousand Gold Prescriptions (Qian Jin Fang, 千金方)* by Sun, Si-miao (孫思邈) described the method of leading qi and also described the use of the six sounds. The use of the six sounds to regulate qi in the internal organs had already been used by the Buddhists and Daoists for some time. Sun, Si-miao also introduced a massage system called Lao Zi's 49 Massage Techniques. *The Extra Important Secret (Wai Tai Mi Yao, 外台秘要)* by Wang, Tao (王燾) discussed the use of breathing and herbal therapies for disorders of qi circulation.

During the Song, Jin, and Yuan dynasties (宋, 金, 元) (AD 960–1368), *Life Nourishing Secrets (Yang Shen Jue, 養生訣)* by Zhang, An-dao (張安道) discussed several qigong practices. *The Confucian Point of View (Ru Men Shi Shi, 儒門視事)* by Zhang, Zi-he (張子和) uses qigong to cure external injuries such as cuts and sprains. *Secret Library of the Orchid Room (Lan Shi Mi Cang, 蘭室秘藏)* by Li, Guo (李果) uses qigong and herbal remedies for internal disorders. *A Further Thesis of Complete Study (Ge Zhi Yu Lun, 格致餘論)* by Zhu, Dan-xi (朱丹溪) provided a theoretical explanation for the use of qigong in curing disease.

During the Song dynasty (宋) (AD 960–1279), not long after the Shaolin temple started using qigong in their martial training, Zhang, San-feng (張三豐) is believed to have created taijiquan. Taiji follows a different approach in its use of qigong than does

Shaolin. While Shaolin emphasizes external elixir (*wai dan*, 外丹) qigong exercises, taiji emphasizes internal elixer (*nei dan*, 內丹) qigong training. (See the next section for wai dan and nei dan).

In AD 1026, the famous brass man of acupuncture was built by Dr. Wang, Wei-yi (王維一). Before this time, there were many publications that discussed acupuncture theory, principles, and treatment techniques, but there were many disagreements among them, and many points that were unclear. When Dr. Wang built his brass man, he also wrote a book called *Illustration of the Brass Man Acupuncture and Moxibustion (Tong Ren Yu Xue Zhen Jiu Tu*, 銅人俞穴鍼灸圖). He explained the relationship of the twelve organs and the twelve qi channels, clarified many of the points of confusion, and for the first time systematically organized acupuncture theory and principles. In AD 1034, he used acupuncture to cure the emperor Ren Zong (仁宗). With the support of the emperor, acupuncture flourished. Ren Zong's work contributed greatly to the advancement of qigong and Chinese medicine by giving a clear and systematic idea of the circulation of qi in the human body.

Later, in the Southern Song dynasty (南宋) (AD 1127–1279), Marshal Yue, Fei (岳飛) was credited with creating several internal qigong exercises and martial arts. It is said that the Eight Pieces of Brocade (*Ba Duan Jin*, 八段錦) was created by Marshal Yue, Fei to improve his soldiers' health. He was also known as the creator of the internal martial style *Xingyi* (形意). In addition to that, Eagle Style martial artists also claim that Yue, Fei was the creator of their style.

From then until the end of the Qing dynasty (清) (AD 1911), many other qigong styles were founded. The well-known ones include Tiger Step Gong (*Hu Bu Gong*, 虎步功), Twelve Postures (*Shi Er Zhuang*, 十二庄), and Beggar Gong (*Jiao Hua Gong*, 叫化功). Also in this period, many documents related to qigong were published, such as *The Secret Important Document of Body Protection (Bao Shen Mi Yao*, 保身祕要) by Cao, Yuan-bai (曹元白), which described moving and stationary qigong practice; *Brief Introduction to Nourishing the Body (Yang Sheng Fu Yu*, 養生膚語) by Chen, Ji-ru (陳繼儒), about the three treasures: essence (*jing*, 精), internal energy (*qi*, 氣), and spirit (*shen*, 神). Also, *The Total Introduction to Medical Prescriptions (Yi Fang Ji Jie*, 醫方集介), by Wang, Fan-an (汪汎庵), reviewed and summarized the previously published materials; and *Illustrated Explanation of Nei Gong (Nei Gong Tu Shuo*, 內功圖說) by Wang, Zu-yuan (王祖元), which presented the Twelve Pieces of Brocade and also explained the idea of combining both moving and stationary qigong.

In the late Ming dynasty (明) (AD 1640) a martial qigong style, Fire Dragon Gong (*Huo Long Gong*, 火龍功) was created by the *Taiyang* (太陽宗) martial stylists. Late in the Qing dynasty (清) (AD 1644–1911), the well-known internal martial art style named *Baguazhang* (八卦掌) was created by Dong, Hai-chuan (董海川) (AD 1797–1882). This style is now gaining in popularity throughout the world.

Before 1911, Chinese society was still very old fashioned and conservative. Even though China had been expanding its contact with the outside world for the last hundred years, the outside world had little influence beyond the coastal regions. With the overthrow of the Qing dynasty and the founding of the Chinese Republic, the nation started changing as never before. Therefore, we would like to draw a line at 1911 and consider the time since then as a new period. Before we discuss the present period, let us first summarize a few points that marked the characteristics of the previous period:

1. Qigong was adapted into the martial arts, and martial qigong styles were created.

2. Qi circulation theory and Chinese acupuncture technologies had reached a peak. More documents were published about medical qigong than about regular qigong exercises.

3. Religious qigong practice remained secret.

4. Qigong exercises had become more popular in Chinese society.

### From the Late Qing Dynasty to the Present

Since 1911, qigong practice has entered a new era. Because of the ease of communication in the modern world, Western culture is having a great influence on the Orient. Many Chinese have opened their minds and changed their traditional ideas, especially in Taiwan and Hong Kong. The various qigong styles are now being taught openly, and many formerly secret documents have been published. Modern methods of communication have opened qigong to a much wider audience than ever before, and people now have the chance to study and understand many different styles. In addition, people are now able to compare Chinese qigong to similar arts from other countries such as India, Japan, Korea, and the Middle East. I deeply believe that in the near future qigong will be considered the most exciting and challenging field of research. It is an ancient science just waiting to be investigated with the help of the new technologies now being developed at an almost explosive rate. Anything we can do to speed up this research will greatly help humanity to understand and improve itself.

## 1-4. History of the Eight Pieces of Brocade

The Eight Pieces of Brocade were created by Marshal Yue, Fei (岳飛) to improve the health of his soldiers. It is said that originally, there were twelve pieces of brocade, but after being passed down from generation to generation for more than eight hundred years, they were edited down to eight pieces. Yue, Fei is not only credited with being the creator of the Eight Pieces of Brocade, but he is also recognized as the founder of two martial styles: Eagle Claw (*Yingzhua*, 鷹爪), an external style, and *Xingyi* (形意), an internal style. Yue, Fei is considered one of the wisest and bravest heroes in the history of

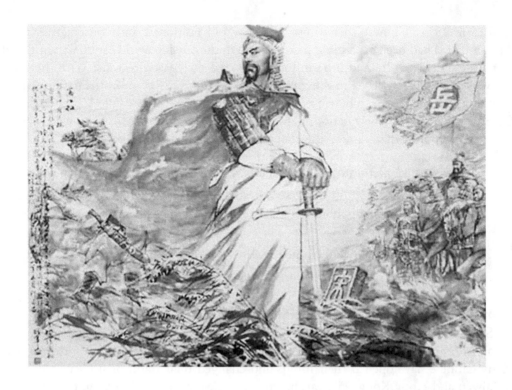

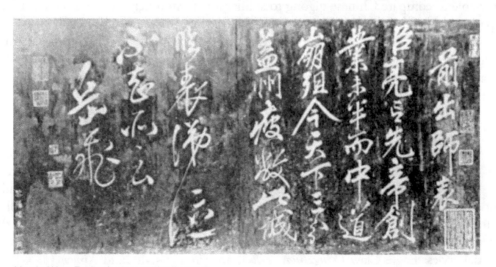

Marshal Yue, Fei (top), stone tablet (bottom).

China, and he is highly respected even today. Before you start practicing this set of qigong exercises, from which the Chinese people have benefitted for nearly one thousand years, it is good to first study the background of its creator.

The Song dynasty in China was a sorrowful time for the Chinese. Wars with the northern barbarians, the Jin race (金), corruption in business and government, and the specter of starvation constantly oppressed the people. Nevertheless, in the midst of all these troubles there arose a man who showed by the purity of his spirit and ideals that goodness, righteousness, and loyalty were qualities that still lived. For countless generations after his betrayal and murder at the hands of traitors, Marshal Yue, Fei remains the ideal for the Chinese people of the completely virtuous man. In peace, Yue, Fei was a great scholar of the Chinese classics. In war, Yue, Fei was a brave and shrewd general who skillfully defeated the enemies of his country.

Yue, Fei was born on February 15, 1103 AD, in Tang Yin Xian (湯陰縣), Henan Province (河南省). While he was being born, a momentous event took place: a large, powerful bird called a roc (*peng*, 鵬) flew onto the roof and began to make a tremendous noise. The father sensed that the bird's presence was an omen that foretold a tumultuous yet inspired fate for his son; the father thus named his son Fei, which in Chinese means "to fly." This reflected the father's belief that his son would fly to great and noble heights as a man.

When Yue, Fei was but one month old, tragedy struck: the Yellow River flooded. Yue, Fei's mother saved herself and her infant son by taking refuge in a giant urn; the urn acted as a small boat and took both mother and son to safety. When they reached dry land and the flood had receded, they went back to find that their home and property were totally destroyed.

Yue, Fei's mother was very poor, but she was a well-educated scholar and possessed the courage, intelligence, and bravery to raise her son properly while giving him noble ideals. Because they were too poor to pay for an education, Yue, Fei's mother taught him personally. Each day she taught him how to read and write by drawing figures in the sand. Even though other children had books, paper, and brushes, the poor Yue, Fei became one of the most educated youngsters in his village; few children could match his scholarship.

In many ways the most important person and the greatest influence on Yue, Fei's life was his mother. All the ideals that Yue, Fei lived and died for were taught to him by his mother. They held their own classes using the sand as a blackboard. Without his mother's teachings and example, Yue, Fei would never have become the brave, intelligent, and loyal leader that he was.

The young Yue, Fei was an avid reader. His favorite subjects were history and military theory. The book he admired and studied the most was *Sun's Book of Tactics (Sun Zi Bing Fa*, 孫子兵法*)*, a book written by Sun, Wu (孫武, c. 557 BC) describing the theory and practice of warfare. From this book Yue learned important principles that later helped him in his military career.

When Yue, Fei was a young man, he became a tenant farmer for a landlord named Han, Qi (韓琦). After long hours of work, he would come home to continue studying with his mother. Yue, Fei was much admired for this and for the great physical st,rength he showed as a young man. As in scholarship, no one could match his natural power and speed.

These admirable qualities were noticed by a certain man in the town called Zhou, Tong (周侗). Zhou, Tong himself was a scholar and a very good martial artist who had studied in the Shaolin temple. Seeing that Yue, Fei possessed many noble qualities, Zhou, Tong began to teach him martial arts. Martial arts as it was taught to Yue, Fei was a complete system involving bare hand combat, weapons, military tactics, horsemanship, archery, and other related subjects. Through constant practice, Yue, Fei mastered everything Zhou, Tong taught him.

When Yue, Fei was nineteen years old, AD 1122, he decided to aid his country by joining the Song army in its war against the Jin, a nomadic people who had invaded the country. The Song dynasty, which was originally located in northern China, had to move to the south to reestablish itself with a new capital and emperor because the Jin had sacked their old capital and captured their emperor. The Song dynasty, which was invaded, is known as the Northern Song (AD 960–1127), while the Song dynasty that established itself in the south after the Jin invasion is known as the Southern Song (AD 1127–1279). For years, the weakened Southern Song had to pay tribute to the Jin to keep them from attacking farther south. When Yue, Fei joined the army, the Southern Song was trying to regain its lost land by war.

Yue, Fei proved himself to be an extraordinary soldier. His wisdom, bravery, and martial skill earned him promotion after promotion so that he became a general after only six years. Later, Yue, Fei became the commander or marshal of the army that was assigned to fight the Jin. Upon assuming command, he instituted a systematic training program in martial arts for his soldiers. Although some martial training had previously existed, Yue, Fei was the first to introduce martial techniques, (*wushu,* 武術), into the army as a basic requirement before combat. Many times a young man joined the army only to find himself in battle the very next day. After a while, Yue's troops, known as Yue Family Troop (*Yue Jia Jun,* 岳家軍) became a highly efficient and successful fighting unit.

The success of Yue's troops can basically be attributed to three things. First, he made all his training strict; the troops were trained in a serious and professional manner. The soldiers were pushed until they excelled in martial arts. Second, Yue, Fei set up a military organization that was efficient and well run. Third, and most important, Yue, Fei created for his troops two new styles of wushu. The first style that he taught to the troops came from his internal training and led to the creation of Xingyi (形意). The second style, which he created out of external wushu, was Eagle Claw, a style that put a major emphasis on *qin na* (擒拿).

With his highly trained troops, Yue, Fei was in favor of pressing the attack against the Jin. He was so loyal and patriotic that he felt it was shameful for the Song to pay the Jin tribute. Yue, Fei constantly felt intense personal agony from the humiliation that his country suffered. With the desire to free his country constantly on his mind, Yue, Fei on his own initiative advanced his troops against the Jin to win back honor for the Song.

When Yue, Fei went into battle, his highly trained troops had many victories as they began to march north. But Yue, Fei had not yet encountered the Jin commander Wu Zhu (兀朮), who had never lost a battle. Wu Zhu's terrifying success was largely due to his main weapon—the feared *guai zi ma* (枴子馬). The guai zi ma was an ancient version of the tank. It was a chariot carrying armored men, drawn by three fully armored horses that were connected by a chain. It was extremely difficult to disable either the horses or the riders, and so they completely dominated the battlefield.

Yue, Fei had given much thought to defending against the awful guai zi ma. As in other cases, Yue's brilliant military mind came up with a solution. He found that the horses were not protected in one place—their legs; putting armor on the horses' legs would have made them immobile. It was too difficult to attack the horses' legs by conventional arrows and spears, so Yue, Fei devised two simple but effective weapons: a sword with a hooked end, which was extremely sharp, on the inside edge of the hook, and a shield made out of a vine called "rattan" (*teng*, 藤). This army was called *Teng Pai Jun* (籐牌軍), or "The Rattan Shield Army."

At last, both generals met on a fateful day. When the battle started, Yue, Fei had the Rattan Shield Army crouching very low in the path of the guai zi ma. Before the chariots could reach the soldiers, they ran into obstacles such as ditches and upright spears, which Yue, Fei had set up. Once these slowed down the chariots, Yue, Fei's soldiers, who were mainly on foot, could move against the enemy with more ease. As the chariots advanced, the crouching men hooked and cut the legs of the horses, making them fall. It was impossible for the horses to trample the crouching men because their shields were greased, and the horses slipped every time they put their feet on them. When the crouching soldiers attacked the horses, they had to cripple only one animal to stop a chariot. Once a chariot was stopped, other Yue, Fei soldiers surrounded it and killed the riders. On that day, Yue, Fei scored a military victory that lives today in history and legend.

Yue, Fei then proceeded north, regaining lost territory and defeating such Jin generals as the Tiger King and the Great Dragon. However, while Yue, Fei was regaining his country's honor, the Jin leaders successfully bribed one of the most infamous men in

Chinese history—Qin, Kuai (秦檜)—to stop Yue, Fei. Qin, Kuai was at that time the prime minister and the most influential man at the emperor's corrupt court.

While Yue, Fei's army moved north, Qin, Kuai, to achieve his evil act, decided to send an imperial order with the emperor's official golden seal (*jin pai*, 金牌), asking Yue, Fei to come back. According to tradition, a general fighting on the front line had the option of refusing an order of retreat. Qin, Kuai was counting on Yue, Fei's patriotic sense of loyalty to the emperor to get him back. To ensure Yue, Fei's return, Qin, Kuai sent twelve gold-sealed orders in one day; so much pressure made Yue, Fei return.

When Yue, Fei returned, he was immediately imprisoned. Because Qin, Kuai feared that any sort of trial would reveal Yue, Fei's innocence, he ordered an officer named He, Zhu (何鑄) to thoroughly investigate Yue, Fei's life in an attempt to find some excuse for the imprisonment. He, Zhu searched and searched, but he found nothing. Although a powerful general, Yue, Fei had never abused his position for bad purposes. He, Zhu found that Yue, Fei had lived a spartan life and had fewer possessions than a peasant. When He, Zhu returned to Qin, Kuai, he reported only one fact of significance. When Yue, Fei joined the army his mother tattooed on his back a certain phrase: "Be Loyal and Pure to Serve Your Country" (*Jing Zhong Bao Guo*, 精忠報國).

With such an honest general as Yue, Fei, Qin, Kuai had only one alternative—to have his food poisoned. Thus was the noble general viciously betrayed by his own countryman. Without the glory and honor that was his right, Yue, Fei died in jail on January 27, 1142, December 9, 1141 on the Chinese calendar. Yue, Fei was thirty-eight years old. Later, Yue, Fei's adopted son, Yue, Yun (岳雲), and Yue, Fei's top assistant, Zhang, Xian (張憲), were also killed.

For more than twenty years, Yue, Fei was officially considered a criminal. But in AD 1166 a new and better government and emperor, Xiao, Zong (孝宗), took control. He refused to believe in the treachery of Yue, Fei and relocated his grave to the beautiful West Lake in Hangzhou (杭州。西湖). In front of the grave are stone statues of Qin, Kuai and his wife, kneeling in repentance and shame before Yue, Fei. These statues have to be replaced periodically because many of the people who come to worship at the grave will deface or damage them out of anger at their treachery. Emperor Xiao Zong bestowed upon Yue, Fei a new name, which symbolized what he always was and always will be—Yue, Wu Mu (岳武穆)—"Yue, the righteous and respectable warrior."

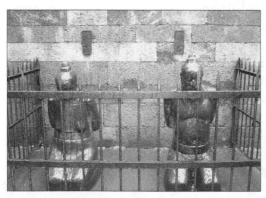

Stone statues of Qin, Kuai and his wife.

## 1-5. Qigong Theory and Training Categories

Many people think that qigong is a difficult subject to understand. In some ways, this is true. However, you must understand one thing: regardless of how difficult the qigong theory and practice of a particular style are, the basic theory and principles are very simple and remain the same for all of the qigong styles. The basic theory and principles are the roots of the entire qigong practice. If you understand these roots, you will be able to grasp the key of the practice and grow. All of the qigong styles originated from this root, but each one has blossomed differently.

In this section, we will discuss these basic theories and principles. With this knowledge as a foundation, you will be able to understand not only what you should be doing, but also why you are doing it. Naturally, it is impossible to discuss all of the basic qigong ideas in such a short section. However, it will offer the beginner the key to open the gate into the spacious, four-thousand-year-old garden of Chinese qigong.

### Qi and Humans

In order to use qigong to improve and maintain your health, you must know that there is qi in your body, and you must understand how it circulates and what you can do to insure that the circulation is smooth and strong.

After reading the above discussion, you know that qi is energy. It is a requirement for life. The qi in your body cannot be seen, but it can be felt. This qi can make your body feel too positive (*yang,* 陽) or too negative (*yin,* 陰).

Imagine that your physical body is a machine, and your qi is the current that makes it run. Without the current, the machine is dead and unable to function. It is the same with qi in your body. For example, when you pinch yourself, you feel pain. Have you ever thought, "How do I feel pain?" You might answer that it is because you have a nervous system in your body that perceives the pinch and sends a signal to the brain. However, you should understand that there is more to it than that. The nervous system is material, and if it didn't have energy circulating in it, it wouldn't function. Qi is the energy that makes the nervous system and the other parts of your body work. When you pinch your skin, that area is stimulated and the qi field is disturbed. Your brain is designed to sense this and other disturbances, and to interpret the cause.

The qi in your body is divided into two categories: managing qi (*ying qi,* 營氣), which is often called nutritive qi, and guardian qi (*wei qi,* 衛氣). The managing qi is the energy that has been sent to the organs so that they can function. The guardian qi is the energy that has been sent to the surface of the body to form a shield to protect you from negative outside influences such as colds. In order to keep yourself healthy, you must learn how to manage these two qi's efficiently so they can serve you well.

How does qi circulate in the body? Chinese doctors discovered long ago that the human body has twelve major channels and eight vessels through which the qi circulates. The twelve channels are like rivers that distribute qi throughout the body and also connect the extremities (fingers and toes) to the internal organs. We would like to point out here that the "internal organs" of Chinese medical theory do not necessarily correspond to the physical organs as understood in the West, but rather to a set of clinical functions similar to each other, and related to the organ system. The eight vessels, which are often referred to as the extraordinary vessels, function like reservoirs and regulate the distribution and circulation of qi in your body.

When the qi in the eight reservoirs is full and strong, the qi in the rivers is strong and will be regulated efficiently. When there is stagnation in any of these twelve channels or rivers, the qi that flows to the body's extremities and to the internal organs will be abnormal, and illness may develop. You should understand that every channel has its particular qi flow strength, and every channel is different. All of these different levels of qi strength are affected by your mind, the weather, the time of day, the food you have eaten, and even your mood. For example, when the weather is dry, the qi in the lungs will tend to be more positive than when it is moist. When you are angry, the qi flow in your liver channel will be abnormal. The qi strength in the different channels varies throughout the day in a regular cycle, and at any particular time, one channel is strongest. For example, between 11 a.m. and 1 p.m. the qi flow in the heart channel is the strongest. Furthermore, the qi level of the same organ can be different from one person to another.

Whenever the qi flow in the twelve rivers or channels is not normal, the eight reservoirs will regulate the qi flow and bring it back to normal. For example, when you experience a sudden shock, the qi flow in the bladder immediately becomes deficient. Now, normally the reservoir will immediately regulate the qi in this channel so that you recover from the shock. However, if the reservoir qi is also deficient, or if the effect of the shock is too great and there is not enough time to regulate the qi, the bladder will suddenly contract, causing unavoidable urination.

When a person is sick because of an injury, his qi level tends to be either too positive (excessive) yang, or too negative (deficient) yin. A Chinese physician would either use a prescription of herbs to adjust the qi, or else he would insert acupuncture needles at various spots on the channels to inhibit the flow in some channels and stimulate the flow in others, so that balance can be restored. However, there is another alternative and that is to use certain physical and mental exercises to adjust the qi. In other words, use qigong.

## Qigong Categories

As you can see, it is very important to keep the qi or internal energy circulating smoothly in your body. Many different kinds of qigong exercises have been created to achieve this, but they can generally be categorized into five groups according to the main purpose of the training:

### 1. Maintaining Health

The main purpose of the qigong styles in this category is to first gain mental and spiritual calmness, peace, and balance. With this mental balance, you can then engage in moving exercises that maintain the smoothness and balance of the qi circulation. This category uses both still meditation and moving meditative exercises.

It is believed that many illnesses are caused by mental and emotional excesses. These emotions use up qi and cause stagnation in the channels and organ systems, which causes you to get sick. For example, depression can cause stomach ulcers and indigestion. Anger will cause the liver to malfunction. Sadness will cause compression and tightness in the lungs, and fear can disturb the normal functioning of the kidneys and bladder. Chinese qigong practitioners therefore realized that if you want to avoid illness, the first step is to balance and relax your thoughts. This is called "regulating the mind" (*tiao xin*, 調心). When your mind is calm and you are emotionally neutral, your qi will automatically regulate itself and correct imbalances.

In the still meditation used for maintaining health, a major part of the training is getting rid of thoughts so that the mind is clear and calm. When you become peaceful and calm, the flow of thoughts and emotions slows down, and you feel mentally and emotionally neutral. This kind of meditation can be thought of as practicing emotional self-control. When you are in this "no thought" state, you become very relaxed and can even relax deep down into your internal organs. When your body is this relaxed, your qi will naturally flow smoothly and strongly, clearing obstructions in the channels and maintaining your health. This kind of still meditation was very common in ancient Chinese scholarly society.

Chinese physicians discovered that certain movements or exercises increased the qi circulation around the internal organs. Some of these movements are similar to movements that are characteristic of certain animals. It is clear that in order for an animal to survive in the wild, it must have an instinct for how to protect its body. Part of this instinct is concerned with how to build up its qi and how to keep its qi from being lost. We humans have lost many of these instincts over the years that we have been separating ourselves from nature. One typical set of these qigong exercises, which is still practiced today, is called Five Animal Sports (Wu Qin Xi, 五禽戲). Another is the Eight Pieces of Brocade.

Over the thousands of years of observing nature and themselves, some qigong practitioners went even deeper. They realized the body's qi circulation changes with the seasons, and it is a good idea to help the body out in these periodic adjustments. They also noticed that during each season, different organs had characteristic problems. For example, in the beginning of autumn your lungs have to adapt to the colder and drier air you are breathing. While this adjustment takes place, the lungs are susceptible to disturbance, so your lungs may feel uncomfortable and you may catch colds easily.

Your digestive system is also affected during seasonal changes. Your appetite may increase, or you may have diarrhea. When the temperature goes down, your kidneys and bladder will start to give you trouble. For example, because the kidneys are stressed, you may feel pain in your back. Focusing on these seasonal qi disorders, the meditators created a set of movements that can be used to speed up the body's adjustment. These qigong exercises will be introduced in a later volume.

### 2. Curing Sickness

Chinese doctors discovered through experience that some of the movements could not only maintain health, but could also cure certain illnesses. Using their medical knowledge of qi circulation, they researched until they had found many movements that could help cure various illnesses and health problems. Naturally, many of them were not unlike the ones used to maintain health. This is not surprising, since many illnesses are caused by unbalanced qi. When this stagnation continues for a long period of time, the organs will start to be affected and may be physically damaged. As a matter of fact, as long as your sickness is limited to the level of qi stagnation and there is no physical organ damage, the qigong exercises used for maintaining health can be used to readjust your qi circulation and treat the problem.

However, if the sickness is already so serious that the physical organs start to fail, then the situation has become critical. In this case, a specific treatment is necessary. The treatment can be acupuncture, herbs, or even an operation. Some qigong exercises are designed to speed up the healing, or sometimes even to cure the sickness. For example, ulcers and asthma can be cured with some simple exercises. Recently in both Mainland China and Taiwan, certain qigong exercises have been shown to be effective in treating certain kinds of cancer.[1]

Acupressure or qigong massage is also commonly used instead of needles to adjust the qi imbalance. This is done mostly by qigong experts who are able to use their body's qi to adjust the patient's qi through touch or acupressure. This is seen in Chinese qigong healing practices and Japanese Shiatsu massage.

### 3. Prolonging Life

The two preceding categories either maintain the health that a person already has, or else treat illnesses once they appear. The theories and the principles for these categories are simple, and the training is conservative. Many Chinese qigong practitioners were not satisfied with this and searched for a way that would not only maintain health, but would also increase the qi circulation and strengthen the organs. In this more aggressive approach to qigong, they attempted to find a way to overcome the normal course of nature. They refused to accept that the length of a person's life is set according to destiny. They believed that if they understood the course of nature (Dao, 道) completely, they would be able to find a way to lengthen their lives. This category of qigong training is practiced mostly by Buddhists and Daoists.

Over the more than nineteen hundred years of research, the religious meditators discovered the way to slow down the degeneration of the organs, which is the key to obtaining a long life. There have been many Buddhists and Daoists who have lived more than 150 years. In Daoist society, it is said: "One hundred and twenty means dying young."[2]

Unfortunately, all of this qigong training has been passed down secretly in the monasteries. Starting in the 1960s, these secret theories and training methods were slowly revealed to the outside world. An important part of this training to prolong life is Marrow/Brain Washing Qigong. The basic idea of Marrow/Brain Washing Qigong is to keep the qi circulating in your marrow and brain so that the marrow and the brain stay fresh and healthy.

Your bone marrow manufactures most of your blood cells. The blood cells bring nourishment to the organs and all the other cells of the body, and also take waste products away. When your blood is healthy and functions properly, your whole body is well-nourished and healthy, and can resist disease effectively. When the marrow is clean and fresh, it manufactures an enormous number of healthy blood cells, which will do their job properly. Your whole body will stay healthy and the organs will not degenerate.

Although the theory is simple, the training is very difficult. You must first learn how to build up your qi and fill up your eight qi vessels, and then you must know how to lead this qi into the bone marrow to "wash" the marrow. However, except for Daoist and Buddhist monks, there are very few people who have lived more than 150 years. The reason for this is that the training process is long and hard. You must have a pure mind and a simple lifestyle so that you can concentrate entirely on the training. Without a peaceful life, your training will not be effective. This is why the Daoist and Buddhist monks hide themselves in the mountains. Unfortunately, this is simply not possible for the average person.

**4. Martial Arts**

In the Liang dynasty (梁), martial artists started to use qigong to increase the effectiveness of their arts. Such training can also help to improve health. However, some martial artists will even use certain qigong practices which they know will harm their health, if these practices will improve some aspect of their fighting ability. An example of this kind of training is iron sand palm.

**5. Enlightenment or Buddhahood**

The Daoists and Buddhists use qigong to reach a level of attainment far beyond the average person's. They are striving for enlightenment, or what the Buddhists refer to as Buddhahood. They are looking for a way to lift themselves above normal human suffering and to escape from the cycle of continual reincarnation. In order to reach this stage, Marrow/Brain Washing Qigong training is necessary. This enables them to lead qi to the forehead, where the spirit resides, and raise the brain to a higher energy state. This is discussed more deeply in the book, *Qigong—The Secret of Youth,* available from YMAA Publication Center.

## 1-6. Qigong Training

Generally speaking, all qigong practices, according to theory and training, can be divided into two general categories: external elixir (wai dan, 外丹) and internal elixir (nei dan, 內丹). In this section, we will discuss the theories of these two categories. Once you understand these theories, you have the root of most Chinese qigong practices.

### External Elixir (Wai Dan, 外丹)

As previously mentioned, the human body has twelve major qi channels (jing, 經), which can be compared to rivers. Six of these are connected to the fingers, and the other six are connected to the toes. All of these twelve are connected to the internal organs. The body also has eight qi vessels (*mai*, 脈), which serve as reservoirs and regulate the qi in the channels. Millions of tiny channels (*luo*, 絡) carry qi from the major channels to every part of the body, from the skin to the bone marrow. Whenever the qi is stagnant in any of the twelve major channels, the related organ will receive an incorrect amount of qi. This will cause the organ to malfunction, or at least to degenerate sooner than normal, and this in turn will cause illness and premature aging. Just as a machine needs the correct amount of current to run properly, your organs must have the right amount of qi to function well. Therefore, the most basic way to maintain the health of the organs is to keep the qi flow strong and smooth. This is the idea upon which external elixer (wai dan) qigong is based.

The theory is very simple. When you do the wai dan exercises, you concentrate your attention on your limbs. As you exercise, the qi builds up in your arms and legs. When the qi potential in your limbs builds to a high enough level, the qi will flow through the channels, clearing any obstructions and nourishing the organs. This is the main reason that a person who works out or has a physical job is generally healthier than someone who sits all day.

There are many available wai dan qigong sets. A typical one is Da Mo's *Muscle/Tendon Changing Classic* (*Yi Jin Jing*, 易筋經). In this set, the practitioner slightly tenses the local limb muscles, such as in the wrists, and then relaxes completely. Through this repeated tensing and relaxing, the qi is built up to a higher concentration. When the practitioner finishes the exercise and relaxes, the accumulated qi flows back to the organs.

There are other wai dan sets that, in addition to tensing and relaxing the muscles, also move the arms and legs into specific positions so that the muscles around certain organs are also stretched and then relaxed. This increases the qi circulation around and in the organs more directly than the *Muscle/Tendon Changing Classic* does. For example, you may repeatedly raise your arms over your head and then lower them. This extends and stretches the muscles around the lungs. This extension and release gently massages the lungs and stimulates the qi and blood flow there. A typical set of wai dan that uses both stationary and moving exercises is the Eight Pieces of Brocade.

Many qigong beginners mistakenly believe that since wai dan qigong theory and training are simple, these sets are only for beginners. However, most people who train internal elixir (nei dan, 內丹) qigong later come back to wai dan and combine the two to increase their control over their qi. An example of this is taiji qigong. While sitting meditation is purely nei dan, the movements of the taiji solo sequence and the qigong sets are a combination of both nei dan and wai dan.

### Internal Elixir (Nei Dan, 內丹)

In the higher levels of qigong practice, the theory and principles are more difficult to understand. It is not just that the training is harder. Another problem is that the nei dan qigong practices have been passed down more secretly than the wai dan. When nei dan practice reached to the highest level such as Marrow/Brain Washing Qigong, it was passed down only to a few disciples. There are a number of reasons for this:

1. Nei dan is hard to understand, so only the disciples who were intelligent and wise enough to understand it were taught.

2. Nei dan practice can be dangerous. Inaccurate practice may cause crippling, paralysis, or even death. This can happen especially to the disciple who does not understand the what, why, and how of the practice.

3. In most of the nei dan qigong training a disciple must learn and experience directly from a master. Qigong is learned and practiced from feeling and sensation. This feeling must be obtained from a master. If the practitioner tries to figure it out by himself, he may possibly get lost. In some cases, he may even cause his own death.

4. In order to reach the higher levels of nei dan qigong, you must conserve your essence (jing, 精) and restrain your sex life. You must also spend a lot of time in practice, which makes normal married life impossible. Not only that, in order to reach spiritual balance, you must train yourself to be emotionally neutral and independent. In ancient times, in order to preserve your essence (jing) and have a peaceful environment for your training, you almost had to go away to the mountains and become a hermit, or else become a monk in a monastery.

Even though nei dan is difficult to understand and practice, it is still practiced by many non-priests and qigong practitioners in the everyday environment. However, they can only reach a certain level of achievement.

Generally speaking, nei dan is a qigong practice in which the qi is built up inside the body first, and then spread out to the limbs. Nei dan can be broken down into several categories according to the purpose and depth of training. Generally, after the qi is built up internally, a nei dan qigong practitioner will circulate the qi throughout his body. Nei dan includes three paths of qi circulation: fire, wind, and water.

### The Fire Path (Huo Lu, 火路)

The fire path in qigong is the most fundamental nei dan practice among the three. This path is used both by qigong practitioners and martial artists. In the fire path, a practitioner usually builds his qi in the field of elixir (*lower dan tian*, 下丹田) through either abdominal breathing or purely through thinking. When the qi is built up to a level, he will use his mind to lead the qi to circulate through the conception and governing vessels (*ren mai* and *du mai*, 任脈, 督脈). This path starts at the lower dan tian, passes down to the *huiyin* (Co-1, 會陰) and the tailbone, follows the spine up the back, passes over the crown of the head, and moves down the front of the body back to the lower dan tian to complete the cycle. This fire path is the way qi routinely circulates in the average person. When there is excess qi added to this path, there is excess heat (fire).

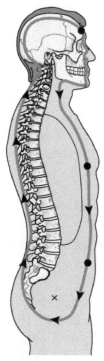

Fire Path.

The conception and governing vessels are two major qi reservoirs that govern or influence the twelve qi channels or rivers. When the qi in these two vessels is strong, the qi circulation in the twelve organ channels will also be strong and thus benefit the body. However, you must understand one thing: the organ qi should not be excessive (yang) or deficient (yin). When too much qi is supplied to the organs, it will overheat the organs and speed their degeneration, just as too much sunshine on your skin will cause it to age faster. Therefore, even though this fire nei dan is the simplest of the three practices, if you are not able to sense your organs' qi level, you might cause problems.

Once a practitioner has opened the circulation path through the conception and governing vessels, he is said to have completed small circulation (*xiao zhou tian*, 小周天). He then leads the qi to the extremities to open the channels in the limbs and also to supply qi to the skin and the bone marrow. When he is able to do this, he has completed large circulation (*da zhou tian*, 大周天).

### The Wind Path (Feng Lu, 風路)

In wind path qi circulation, once the qi is built up in the lower dan tian, the practitioner will lead the qi to circulate in the opposite direction as he did with the fire path. There are many reasons for doing this:

1. To cut down the excess qi circulation (fire) to the internal organs.
2. To slow down the natural qi circulation in the conception and governing vessels if they have become too positive due to sickness, injury, or any other reason.

3. To raise the pre-birth qi, or water qi (jing qi, 精氣) generated in the lower dan tian to cool down the post-birth qi (food and air qi, or fire qi) that is generated in the middle dan tian at the solar plexus. The fire path is the way to do this.

### The Water Path (Shui Lu, 水路)

Water path qigong, which goes through the inside of the spine, is probably one of the highest levels of qigong practice. Once you have built your pre-birth qi in the lower dan tian, you use your mind and special training to lead the qi into the thrusting vessel (*chong mai*, 衝脈), the qi reservoir which is located in the spinal cord. Marrow/Brain Washing Qigong generates qi through a different method than the other forms of qigong. Its approach is to convert semen into qi. The qi that has been generated by either method is led to the brain to energize the brain and spirit (shen, 神). The energized mind is then able to adjust the qi level in the organs and other parts of the body. This qigong practice is difficult to do, but once competence has been achieved it is the most efficient. It is reported that priests who reach this level are able to slow down the aging process to a minimum, and some are able to live over two hundred years.

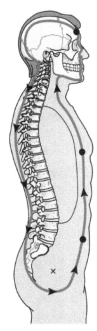

Wind Path.

Marrow/Brain Washing Qigong has been kept top secret within the Daoist and Buddhist societies. Not only does it enable them to live long and healthy lives, but it is also involved with how they work to reach enlightenment or Buddhahood. Enlightenment or Buddhahood is the final goal of a priest who is looking for the eternal spiritual life. If you are interested in more information about Marrow/Brain Washing Qigong, please refer to the book *Qigong—The Secret of Youth,* available from YMAA Publication Center

The water path way enables you to reduce the excess fire, which most people build up. However, the training is the hardest both to practice and to understand.

## Chapter Summary

Before we finish this section, we would like to conclude the discussion with the following thoughts:

1. Wai dan qigong is a practice in which qi is built up in the limbs and then flows to the organs, while in nei dan practice the qi is built up in the body and then spread out to the limbs. Wai dan practice is mostly physical while nei dan practice is primarily mental.

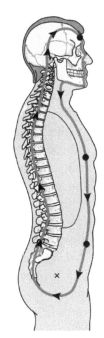

Water Path.

2. Wai dan is commonly done through muscle tension and relaxation exercises. Wai dan can also be done with movement of the limbs. Nei dan can be done either through lower dan tian exercises or simply through thinking.

3. Massage, acupuncture, and acupressure are considered wai dan because they rely on outside assistance to adjust the qi balance.

4. Nei dan can be dangerous while wai dan is usually safe.

Because this book focuses on wai dan qigong, this section serves only as a general introduction, and all of the above discussions have necessarily been brief. Interested readers should refer to other documents and books published by YMAA Publication Center.

## 1-7. How to Use This Book

When you practice any qigong, you must first ask "What," "Why," and "How." "What" means "What am I looking for?" "What do I expect?" and "What should I do?" Then you must ask, "Why do I need it?" "Why does it work?" "Why must I do it this way instead of that way?" Finally, you must determine "How does it work?" "How much have I advanced toward my goal?" and "How will I be able to advance further?"

It is very important to understand what you are practicing, and not just automatically repeat what you have learned. Understanding is the root of any work. With understanding, you will be able to know your goal. Once you know your goal, your mind can be firm and steady. With this understanding, you will be able to see why something has happened and what the principles and theories behind it are. Without all of this, your work will be done blindly, and it will be a long and painful process. Only when you are sure what your target is and why you need to reach it should you raise the question of how you are going to do it. The answers to all of these questions form the root of your practice and will help you avoid the wondering and confusion that uncertainty brings. If you keep this root, you will be able to apply the theory and make it grow—you will know how to create. Without this root, what you learn will be only branches and flowers, and in time they will wither.

In China, there is a story about an old man who was able to change a piece of rock into gold. One day, a boy came to see him and asked for his help. The old man said: "Boy! What do you want? Gold? I can give you all of the gold you want." The boy replied: "No, Master, what I want is not your gold. What I want is the trick!" When you just have gold, you can spend it all and become poor again. If you have the trick of how to make gold, you will never be poor. For the same reason, when you learn qigong you should learn the theory and principle behind it, not just the practice. Understanding theory and principle will not only shorten your time of pondering and practice, but also enable you to practice most efficiently.

One of the hardest parts of the training process is learning how to actually do the forms correctly. Every qigong movement has its special meaning and purpose. In order to make sure your movements or forms are correct, it is best to work with the video and book together. There are some important things that you may not be able to pick up from reading, but once you see them, they will be clear. An example is the transition movements between the forms. Naturally, there are other important ideas which are impossible to take the time to explain in the videotape, such as the theory and principles; these can only be explained in the book. It cannot be denied that under the tutelage of a master you can learn more quickly and perfectly than is possible using only tapes and books. What you are missing is the master's experience. However, if you ponder carefully and practice patiently and perseveringly, you will be able to fill this void through your own experience and practice. This book and the videotape were designed for self-instruction. You will find that they will serve you as a key to enter into the field of qigong.

To conclude, you must practice perseveringly and patiently. You need a strong will and a great deal of patience and self-discipline. You may have already found that there are many different versions of the Eight Pieces of Brocade available on the market. Do not be confused by all of these versions. You should understand that it does not matter which version you practice; the basic theory and principles remain the same. The most important thing of all is to understand the poems and songs that have been passed down through generations. These poems and songs are the root of the training, so please study them carefully.

## References

1. There are many reports in popular and professional literature of using qigong to help or even cure many illnesses, including cancer. Many cases have been discussed in the Chinese qigong journals. One book, which describes the use of qigong to cure cancer, is *New Qigong for Preventing and Curing Cancer* (新氣功防治癌症) by Ye, Ming (葉明), Chinese Yoga Publications, Taiwan, 1986.

2. (一百二十謂之夭。)

# Chapter 2. Qigong Training Theory

## 2-1. Introduction

Before you start your qigong training, you must first understand the three treasures of life: essence (jing, 精), internal energy (qi, 氣), and spirit (shen, 神)—as well as their interrelationship. If you lack this understanding, you are missing the root of qigong training, as well as the basic idea of qigong theory. The main goals of qigong training are to learn how to retain your jing, strengthen and smooth your qi flow, and enlighten your shen. To reach these goals you must learn how to regulate the body (tiao shen, 調身), regulate the mind (tiao xin, 調心), regulate the breathing (*tiao xi*, 調息), regulate the qi (*tiao qi*, 調氣), and regulate the shen (tiao shen, 調神).

Regulating the body includes understanding how to find and build the root of the body as well as of the individual forms you are practicing. To build a firm root, you must know how to keep your center, how to balance your body, and most important of all, how to relax so that the qi can flow.

Regulating the mind involves learning how to keep your mind calm, peaceful, and centered, so that you can judge situations objectively and lead qi to the desired places. The mind is the main key to success in qigong practice.

To regulate your breathing, you must learn how to breathe so that your breathing and your mind mutually correspond and cooperate. When you breathe this way, your mind will be able to attain peace more quickly, and therefore concentrate more easily on leading the qi.

Regulating the qi is one of the ultimate goals of qigong practice. In order to regulate your qi effectively, you must first have regulated your body, mind, and breathing. Only then will your mind be clear enough to sense how the qi is distributed in your body and understand how to adjust it.

For Buddhist priests, who seek the enlightenment of the Buddha, regulating the shen is the final goal of qigong. This enables them to maintain a neutral, objective perspective of life, and this perspective is the eternal life of the Buddha. The average qigong practitioner has lower goals. He raises his shen in order to increase his concentration and enhance his vitality. This makes it possible for him to lead qi effectively to his entire body so that it carries out the managing and guarding duties. This maintains his health and slows down the aging process.

If you understand these few things you will be able to quickly enter into the field of qigong. Without all of these important elements, your training will be ineffective and your time will be wasted.

## 2-2. Three Treasures (Jing, Qi, Shen, 三寶—精，氣，神)

Before you start any qigong training, you must first understand the three treasures (*san bao*, 三寶): essence (jing, 精), internal energy (qi, 氣), and spirit (shen, 神). They are also called the three origins or the three roots (*san yuan*, 三元) because they are considered the origins and roots of your life. Jing means the essence, the most original and refined part of every thing. Jing exists in everything. It represents the most basic part of anything that shows its characteristics. Sperm is called *jing zi* (精子), which means "essence of the son," because it contains the jing of the father, which is passed on to his son (or daughter) and becomes the child's jing. Jing is the original source of every living thing, and it determines the nature and characteristics of that thing. It is the root of life.

Qi is the internal energy of your body. It is like the electricity that passes through a machine to keep it running. Qi comes either from the conversion of the jing that you have received from your parents, or from the food you eat and the air you breathe.

Shen is the center of your mind, the spirit of your being. It is what makes you human because animals do not have a shen. The shen in your body must be nourished by your qi or energy. When your qi is full, your shen will be enlivened.

These three elements are interrelated in a number of ways. Chinese meditators and qigong practitioners believe that the body contains two general types of qi. The first type is called original qi (*yuan qi*, 元氣) or pre-birth qi (*xian tian qi*, 先天氣), and it comes from converted original jing (*yuan jing*, 元精), which you get from your parents at conception. The second type, which is called post-birth qi (*hou tian qi*, 後天氣), is drawn from the jing of the food and air we take in. When this qi flows or is led to the brain, it can energize the shen and soul. This energized and raised shen is able to lead the qi to the entire body.

Each one of these three elements or treasures has its own root. You must know the roots so that you can strengthen and protect your three treasures:

1. There are many kinds of jing that your body requires. Except for the jing that you inherit from your parents, which is called original jing (yuan jing, 元精), all other jings must be obtained from food, air, or even the energy surrounding you. Among all of these jings, original jing is the most important one. It is the root and the seed of your life, and your basic strength. If your parents were strong and healthy, your original jing will be strong and healthy, and you will have a strong foundation on which to grow. The Chinese people believe that in order to stay healthy and live a long life, you must protect and maintain this jing. It is like money that you have

invested in a bank. You can live off the interest for a long time, but if you withdraw the principal and spend it, you will have nothing left.

The root of original jing before your birth was in your parents. After birth this original jing stays in its residence—the kidneys, which are considered the root of your jing. When you keep this root strong, you will have sufficient original jing to supply to your body. Although you cannot increase the amount of jing you have, qigong training can improve the quality of your jing. Qigong can also teach you how to convert your jing into original qi more efficiently and how to use this qi effectively.

2. Qi is converted both from the jing that you have inherited from your parents and from the jing that you draw from the food and air you take in. Qi which is converted from the original jing, which you have inherited, is called original qi (yuan qi, 元氣).[1] Just as original jing is the most important type of jing, original qi is the most important type of qi. It is pure and of high quality, while the qi from food and air may make your body too positive or too negative, depending on how and where you absorb it. When you retain and protect your original jing, you will be able to generate original qi in a pure, continuous stream. As a qigong practitioner, you must know how to convert your original jing into original qi in a smooth, steady stream.

Since your original qi comes from your original jing, they both have the kidneys for their root. When your kidneys are strong, the original jing is strong, and the original qi converted from this original jing will also be full and strong. This qi resides in the lower dan tian in your abdomen. Once you learn how to convert your original jing, you will be able to supply your body with all the qi it needs.

3. Shen is the force that keeps you alive. It has no substance, but it gives expression and appearance to your jing. Shen is also the control tower for the qi. When your shen is strong, your qi is strong and you can lead it efficiently. The root of shen (spirit) is your mind (*yi*, 意) or intention. When your brain is energized and stimulated, your mind will be more aware and you will be able to concentrate more intensely. Also, your shen will be raised. Advanced qigong practitioners believe that your brain must always be sufficiently nourished by your qi. It is the qi that keeps your mind clear and concentrated. With an abundant qi supply, the mind can be energized and can raise the shen and enhance your vitality.

The deeper levels of qigong training include the conversion of jing into qi, which is then led to the brain to raise the shen. This process is called "*huan jing bu nao*" (還精補腦) and means "return the jing to nourish the brain." When qi is led to the head, it stays at the upper dan tian (center of the forehead). The upper dan tian is the residence of shen. Qi and shen are mutually related. When your shen is weak, your qi is weak, and your body will degenerate rapidly. Shen is the headquarters of qi. Likewise, qi supports the shen, energizing it and keeping it sharp, clear, and strong. If the qi in your body is weak, your shen will also be weak.

## 2-3. Qigong Training Theory

In qigong training, you must understand the principle behind everything you are doing. The principle is the root of your practice, and it is this root that brings forth the results you want. The root gives life, while the branches and flowers (results) give only temporary beauty. If you keep the root, you can regrow. If you have just branches and flowers, they will die in a short time.

Every qigong form or practice has its special purpose and theory. If you do not know the purpose and theory, you have lost the root (meaning) of the practice. Therefore, as a qigong practitioner, you must continue to ponder and practice until you understand the root of every set or form.

Before you start training, you must first understand that all of the training originates in your mind. You must have a clear idea of what you are doing, and your mind must be calm, centered, and balanced. This also implies that your feeling, sensing, and judgment must be objective and accurate. This requires emotional balance and a clear mind. This takes a lot of hard work, but once you have reached this level, you will have built the root of your physical training, and your yi will be able to lead your qi throughout your physical body.

As mentioned previously, qigong training includes five important elements: regulating the body, regulating the breath, regulating the mind, regulating the qi, and regulating the spirit (shen). These elements are the foundation of successful qigong practice. Without this foundation, your understanding of qigong and your practice will remain superficial.

### 1. Regulating the Body (Tiao Shen, 調身)

Regulating the body is called "tiao shen" (調身) in Chinese. This means to adjust your body until it is in the most comfortable and relaxed state. This implies that your body must be centered and balanced. If it is not, you will be tense and uneasy, and this will affect the judgment of your yi and the circulation of your qi. In Chinese medical society it is said: "(When) shape (body's posture) is not correct, then the qi will not be smooth. (When) the qi is not smooth, the yi (mind) will not be peaceful. (When) the yi is not peaceful, then the qi is disordered."[2] You should understand that the relaxation of your body originates with your yi. Therefore, before you can relax your body, you must first relax or regulate your mind (yi). This is called "*shen xin ping heng*" (身心平衡), which means "body and heart (mind) balanced." The body and the mind are mutually related. A relaxed and balanced body helps your yi to relax and concentrate. When your yi is at peace and can judge things accurately, your body will be centered, balanced, and relaxed.

**Relaxation**

Relaxation is one of the major keys to success in qigong. You should remember that only when you are relaxed will all your muscles be relaxed and your qi channels open. In order to be relaxed, your yi must first be relaxed and calm. When this yi coordinates with your breathing, your body will be able to relax.

In qigong practice, there are three levels of relaxation. The first level is the external physical relaxation, or postural relaxation. This is a very superficial level, and almost anyone can reach it. It consists of adopting a comfortable stance and avoiding unnecessary strain in how you stand and move. The second level is the relaxation of the muscles and tendons. To do this your yi must be directed deep into the muscles and tendons. This relaxation will help open your qi channels and will allow the qi to sink and accumulate in the lower dan tian.

The final stage is the relaxation that reaches the internal organs and the bone marrow. Remember, only if you can relax deep into your body will your mind be able to lead the qi there. Only at this stage will the qi be able to reach everywhere. Then you will feel transparent—as if your whole body has disappeared. If you can reach this level of relaxation, you will be able to communicate with your organs and use qigong to adjust or regulate the qi disorders that are giving you problems. Not only that, you will be able to protect your organs more effectively, and therefore slow down their degeneration.

**Rooting**

In all qigong practice, it is very important to be rooted. Being rooted means to be stable and in firm contact with the ground. If you want to push a car, you have to be rooted so the force you exert into the car will be balanced by a force into the ground. If you are not rooted, when you push the car you will only push yourself away and not move the car. Your root is made up of your body's root, center, and balance.

Before you can develop your root, you must first relax and let your body "settle." As you relax, the tension in the various parts of your body will dissolve, and you will find a comfortable way to stand. You will stop fighting the ground to keep your body up and will learn to rely on your body's structure to support itself. This lets the muscles relax even more. Since your body isn't struggling to stand up, your yi won't be pushing upward, and your body, mind, and qi will all be able to sink. If you let dirty water sit quietly, the impurities will gradually settle down to the bottom, leaving the water above it clear. In the same way, if you relax your body enough to let it settle, your qi will sink to your lower dan tian and the bubbling well (*yongquan*, K-1, 湧泉) in your feet, and your mind will become clear. Then you can begin to develop your root.

To root your body you must imitate a tree and grow an invisible root under your feet. This will give you a firm root to keep you stable in your training. You should know that your root must be wide as well as deep. Naturally, your yi must grow first because it is the yi that leads the qi. Your yi must be able to lead the qi to your feet and be able to communicate with the ground. Only when your yi can communicate with the ground will your qi be able to grow beyond your feet and enter the ground to build the root. The bubbling well cavity is the gate that enables your qi to communicate with the ground.

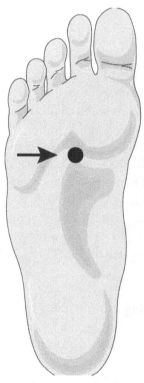

Bubbling well cavity (yongquan, K-1, 湧泉).

After you have gained your root, you must learn how to keep your center. A stable center will make your qi develop evenly and uniformly. If you lose this center, your qi will not be led evenly. In order to keep your body centered, you must first center your yi and then match your body to it. Only under these conditions will the qigong forms you practice have their root. Your mental and physical centers are the keys that enable you to lead your qi beyond your body.

Balance is the product of rooting and centering. Balance includes balancing the qi and the physical body. It does not matter which aspect of balance you are dealing with; first, you must balance your yi, and only then can you balance your qi and your physical body. If your yi is balanced, it can help you to make accurate judgments and therefore to correct the path of the qi flow.

Rooting includes rooting not just the body, but also the form or movement. The root of any form or movement is found in its purpose or principle. For example, in certain qigong exercises you want to lead the qi to your palms. In order to do this, you must imagine that you are pushing an object forward while keeping your muscles relaxed.[3] In this exercise, your elbows must be down to build the sense of root for the push. If you raise the elbows, you lose the sense of "intention" of the movement because the push would be ineffective if you were pushing something for real. Since the intention or purpose of the movement is its reason for being, you now have a purposeless movement, and you have no reason to lead qi in any particular way. Therefore, in this case, the elbow is the root of the movement.

## 2. Regulating the Breath (Tiao Xi, 調息)

Regulating breathing means to regulate your breath until it is calm, smooth, and peaceful. Only when you have reached this point will you be able to make the breathing deep, slender, long, and soft, which is required for successful qigong practice.

Breathing is affected by your emotions. For example, when you are angry, you exhale more strongly than you inhale. When you are sad, you inhale more strongly than you exhale. When your mind is peaceful and calm, your inhalation and exhalation are relatively equal. In order to keep your breathing calm, peaceful, and steady, your mind and emotions must first be calm and neutral. Therefore, in order to regulate your breathing, you must first regulate your mind.

The other side of the coin is that you can use your breathing to control your yi. When your breathing is uniform, it is as if you were hypnotizing your yi, which helps to calm it. From this, you can see that yi and breathing are interdependent and that they cooperate with each other. Deep and calm breathing relaxes you and keeps your mind clear. It fills your lungs with plenty of air, so that your brain and entire body have an adequate supply of oxygen. In addition, deep and complete breathing enables the diaphragm to move up and down, which massages and stimulates the internal organs. For this reason, deep breathing exercises are also called "internal organ exercises."

Deep and complete breathing does not mean that you inhale and exhale to the maximum. This would cause the lungs and the surrounding muscles to tense up, which in turn would keep the air from circulating freely and hinder the absorption of oxygen. Without enough oxygen, your mind becomes scattered, and the rest of your body tenses up. In correct breathing, you inhale and exhale to about 70 percent or 80 percent of capacity, so that your lungs stay relaxed.

You can conduct an easy experiment. Inhale deeply so that your lungs are completely full, and time how long you can hold your breath. Then try inhaling to only about 70 percent of your capacity, and see how long you can hold your breath. You will find that with the latter method you can last much longer than with the first one. This is simply because the lungs and the surrounding muscles are relaxed. When they are relaxed, the rest of your body and your mind can also relax, which significantly decreases your need for oxygen. Therefore, when you regulate your breathing, the first priority is to keep your lungs relaxed and calm.

When training, your mind must first be calm so that your breathing can be regulated. When the breathing is regulated, your mind is able to reach a higher level of calmness. This calmness can again help you to regulate the breathing, until your mind is deep. After you have trained for a long time, your breathing will be full and slender, and your mind will be very clear. It is said: "*xin xi xiang yi*" (心息相依), which means "Heart (mind) and breathing (are) mutually dependent." When you reach this meditative state, your heartbeat slows down and your mind is very clear: you have entered the sphere of real meditation.

An Ancient Daoist named Li, Qing-an (李清菴) said: "Regulating breathing means to regulate the real breathing until (you) stop."[4] This means that correct regulating is no regulating. In other words, although you start by consciously regulating your breath, you must get to the point where the regulating happens naturally, and you no longer have to think about it. When you breathe, if you concentrate your mind on your breathing, then it is not true regulating because the qi in your lungs will become stagnant. When you reach the level of true regulating, no regulating is necessary, and you can use your mind efficiently to lead the qi. Remember, wherever the yi is, there is the qi. If the yi stops in one spot, the qi will be stagnant. It is the yi that leads the qi and makes it move. Therefore, when you are in a state of correct breath regulation, your mind is free. There is no sound, stagnation, urgency, or hesitation, and you can finally be calm and peaceful.

You can see that when the breath is regulated correctly, the qi will also be regulated. They are mutually related and cannot be separated. This idea is explained frequently in Daoist literature. The Daoist Guang Cheng Zi (廣成子) said: "One exhale, the earth qi rises; one inhale, the heaven qi descends; real man's (meaning one who has attained the real Dao) repeated breathing at the navel, then my real qi is naturally connected."[5] This says that when you breathe you should move your abdomen as if you were breathing from your navel. The earth qi is the negative (yin) energy from your kidneys, and the heaven qi is the positive (yang) energy, which comes from the food you eat and the air you breathe. When you breathe from the navel, these two qi's will connect and combine. Some people think that they know what qi is, but they really don't. Once you connect the two qi's, you will know what the "real" qi is, and you may become a "real" man, which means to attain the Dao.

The Daoist book *Sing (of the) Dao (with) Real Words (Chang Dao Zhen Yan,* 唱道真言) says: "One exhale one inhale to communicate qi's function, one movement one calmness is the same as (is the source of) creation and variation."[6] The first part of this statement again implies that the functioning of qi is connected with the breathing. The second part of this sentence means that all creation and variation come from the interaction of movement (yang) and calmness (yin). *Yellow Yard Classic (Huang Ting Jing,* 黃庭經) says: "Breathe original qi to seek immortality."[7] In China, the traditional Daoists wore yellow robes, and they meditated in a "yard" or hall. This sentence means that in order to reach the goal of immortality, you must seek to find and understand the original qi that comes from the lower dan tian through correct breathing.

Moreover, the Daoist Wu Zhen Ren (伍真人) said: "Use the post-birth breathing to look for the real person's (i.e. the immortal's) breathing place."[8] In this sentence, it is clear that in order to locate the immortal breathing place (the lower dan tian), you must rely on and know how to regulate your post-birth, or natural, breathing. Through regulating your post-birth breathing, you will gradually be able to locate the residence of the qi (the lower dan tian), and eventually you will be able to use your lower dan tian to breathe like the immortal Daoists. Finally, in the Daoist song, *The Great Daoist Song of the Spirit's Origin (Ling Yuan Da Dao Ge,* 靈源大道歌) it is said: "The originals (original jing, qi, and shen) are internally transported peacefully, so that you can become real (immortal); (if you) depend (only) on external breathing (you) will not reach the end (goal)."[9] From this song, you can see that internal breathing (breathing at the lower dan tian) is the key to training your three treasures and finally reaching immortality. However, you must first know how to regulate your external breathing correctly.

From the above, you can see the importance of breathing. There are eight key words for air breathing which a qigong practitioner should follow during exercise. Once you understand them, you will be able to substantially shorten the time needed to reach your qigong goals. These eight key words are 1. calm (*jing*, 靜); 2. slender (*xi*, 細); 3. deep (*shen*, 深); 4. long (*chang*, 長); 5. continuous (*you*, 悠); 6. uniform (*yun*, 勻); 7. slow (*huan*, 緩); and 8. soft (*mian*, 綿). These key words are self-explanatory, and with a little thought, you should be able to understand them.

### 3. Regulating the Mind (Tiao Xin, 調心)

It is said in Daoist society: "(When) large Dao is taught, first stop thought; when thought is not stopped, (the lessons are) in vain."[10] This means that when you first practice qigong, the most difficult training is to stop your thinking. The final goal for your mind is "the thought of no thought."[11] Your mind does not think of the past, the present, or the future. Your mind is completely separated from influences of the present such as worry, happiness, and sadness. Then your mind can be calm and steady, and can finally gain peace. Only when you are in the state of "the thought of no thought" will you be relaxed and able to sense calmly and accurately.

Regulating your mind means using your consciousness to stop the activity in your mind in order to set it free from the bondage of ideas, emotion, and conscious thought. When you reach this level, your mind will be calm, peaceful, empty, and light. Then your mind has really reached the goal of relaxation. Only when you reach this stage will you be able to relax deep into your marrow and internal organs. Only then will your mind be clear enough to see (feel) the internal qi circulation and communicate with your qi and organs. In Daoist society it is called "Nei Shi Gongfu" (內視功夫), which means the Gongfu of Internal Vision.

When you reach this real relaxation, you may be able to sense the different elements that make up your body: solid matter, liquids, gases, energy, and spirit. You may even be able to see or feel the different colors that are associated with your five organs: green (liver), white (lungs), black (kidneys), yellow (spleen), and red (heart).

Once your mind is relaxed and regulated and you can sense your internal organs, you may decide to study the five elements theory. This is a very profound subject, and it is sometimes interpreted differently by Oriental physicians and qigong practitioners. When understood properly, it can give you a method of analyzing the interrelationships between your organs and help you devise ways to correct imbalances.

For example, the lungs correspond to the element metal, and the heart to the element fire. Metal (the lungs) can be used to adjust the heat of the fire (the heart) because metal can take a large quantity of heat away from fire, (and thus cool down the heart). When you feel uneasy or have heartburn (excess fire in the heart), you may use deep breathing to calm down the uneasy emotions or cool off the heartburn.

Naturally, it will take a lot of practice to reach this level. In the beginning, you should not have any ideas or intentions because they will make it harder for your mind to relax and empty itself of thoughts. Once you are in a state of "no thought," place your attention on your lower dan tian. It is said, "*yi shou dan tian*" (意守丹田), which means "The mind is kept on the dan tian." The dan tian is the origin and residence of your qi. Your mind can build up the qi at the dan tian, which is called start the fire (*qi huo*, 起火), then lead the qi anywhere you wish, and finally lead the qi back to its residence. When your mind is on the lower dan tian, your qi will always have a root. When you keep this root, your qi will be strong and full, and it will go where you want it to. You can see that when you practice qigong, your mind cannot be completely empty and relaxed. You must find the firmness within the relaxation, and then you can reach your goal.

In qigong training, it is said: "Use your yi (mind) to lead your qi" (*Yi yi yin qi*, 以意引氣). Notice the word "lead." Qi behaves like water—it cannot be pushed, but it can be led. When qi is led, it will flow smoothly and without stagnation. When it is pushed, it will flood and enter the wrong paths. Remember, wherever your yi goes first, the qi will naturally follow. For example, if you intend to lift an object, this intention is your yi. This yi will lead the qi to the arms to energize the muscles, and then the object can be lifted.

It is said: "Your yi cannot be on your qi. Once your yi is on your qi, the qi is stagnant." When you want to walk from one spot to another, you must first mobilize your intention and direct it to the goal; then your body will follow. The mind must always be ahead of the body. If your mind stays on your body, you will not be able to move.

In qigong training, the first thing to know is what qi is. If you do not know what qi is, how will you be able to lead it? Once you know what qi is and experience it, then your yi will have something to lead. The next thing to know is how your yi communicates with your qi. This means that your yi should be able to sense and feel the qi flow and understand how strong and smooth it is. In taiji qigong society, it is commonly said that your yi must "listen" to your qi and "understand" it. Listen means to pay careful attention to what you sense and feel. The more you pay attention, the better you will be able to understand. Only after you understand the qi situation will your yi be able to set up the strategy. In qigong your mind or yi must generate the idea (visualize your intention), which is like an order to your qi to complete a certain mission.

The more your yi communicates with your qi, the more efficiently the qi can be led. For this reason, as a qigong beginner, you must first learn about yi and qi, and also learn how to help them communicate efficiently. Yi is the key in qigong practice. Without this yi, you will not be able to lead your qi, let alone build up the strength of the qi or circulate it throughout your entire body.

Remember, when the yi is strong, the qi is strong, and when the yi is weak, the qi is weak. Therefore, the first step of qigong training is to develop your yi. The first secret of a strong yi is calmness. When you are calm, you can see things clearly and not be disturbed by surrounding distractions. With your mind calm, you will be able to concentrate.

Confucius said: "First you must be calm, then your mind can be steady. Once your mind is steady, then you are at peace. Only when you are at peace, are you able to think and finally gain."[12] This process is also applied in meditation or qigong exercise: calm first, then steady, peace, think, and finally gain. That means when you practice qigong, first you must learn to be calm (emotional calmness). Once calm, you will be able to see what you want and firm your mind (steady). This firm and steady mind is your intention or yi (it is how your yi is generated). Only after you know what you really want will your mind gain peace and be able to relax (emotional and physical relaxation). After you have reached this step, you must then concentrate or think in order to execute your intention. Under this thoughtful and concentrated mind, your qi will follow and you will be able to gain what you wish.

## 4. Regulating the Qi (Tiao Qi, 調心)

Before you can regulate your qi, you must first regulate your body, breath, and mind. If you compare your body to a battlefield, then your mind is like the general who generates ideas and controls the situation, and your breathing is the strategy. Your qi is like the soldiers who are led to various places on the battlefield. All four elements are necessary, and all four must be coordinated with each other if you are to win the war against sickness and aging.

If you want to arrange your soldiers most effectively for battle, you must know which area of the battlefield is most important, and where you are weakest (where your qi is deficient) and need to send reinforcements. If you have more soldiers than you need in one area (excessive qi), then you can send them somewhere else where the ranks are thin. As a general, you must also know how many soldiers are available for the battle, and how many you will need to protect yourself and your headquarters. To be successful, not only do you need good strategy (breathing), but you also need to communicate and understand the situation effectively with your troops, or all of your strategy will be in vain. When your yi (the general) knows how to regulate the body (knows the battlefield), how to regulate the breathing (set up the strategy), and how to effectively regulate the qi (direct your soldiers), you will be able to reach the final goal of qigong training.

In order to regulate your qi so that it moves smoothly in the correct paths, you need more than just efficient yi-qi communication. You also need to know how to generate the qi. If you do not have enough qi in your body, how can you regulate it? In a battle, if you do not have enough soldiers to set up your strategy, you have already lost.

When you practice qigong, you must first train to make your qi flow naturally and smoothly. There are some qigong exercises in which you intentionally hold your yi, and thus qi, in a specific area. As a beginner, however, you should first learn how to make the qi flow smoothly instead of building a qi dam, which is commonly done in external martial qigong training.

In order to make qi flow naturally and smoothly, your yi must first be relaxed. Only when your yi is relaxed will your body be relaxed and the qi channels open for the qi to circulate. Then you must coordinate your qi flow with your breathing. Breathing regularly and calmly will make your yi calm, and allow your body to relax.

### 5. Regulating the Shen (Tiao Shen, 調神)

There is one thing that is more important than anything else in a battle, and that is fighting spirit. You may have the best general, who knows the battlefield well and is also an expert strategist, but if his soldiers do not have a high fighting spirit (morale), he might still lose. Remember, spirit is the center and root of a fight. When you keep this center, one soldier can be equal to ten soldiers. When his spirit is high, a soldier will obey his orders accurately and willingly, and his general will be able to control the situation efficiently. In a battle, in order for a soldier to have this kind of morale, he must know why he is fighting, how to fight, and what he can expect after the fight. Under these conditions, he will know what he is doing and why, and this understanding will raise his spirit, strengthen his will, and increase his patience and endurance.

It is the same with qigong training. In order to reach the final goal of qigong exercise, you must have three fundamental spiritual roots: will, patience, and endurance. You must know why, how, and what. Only then will you be able to be sure of your target and know what you are doing.

Shen, which is the Chinese term for spirit, originates from yi (the general). When shen is strong, the yi is firm. When the yi is firm, shen will be steady and calm. From this, you can see that shen is the mental part of a soldier. When shen is high, the qi is strong and easily directed. When the qi is strong, shen is also strong.

### References

1. Before birth you have no qi of your own, but rather you use your mother's qi. When you are born, you start creating qi from the original jing, which you received from your parents. This qi is called pre-birth qi, as well as original qi. It is also called pre-heaven qi (xian tian qi) because it comes from the original jing which you received before you saw the heavens (which here means sky), i.e., before your birth.
2. 形不正則氣不順，氣不順則意不寧，意不寧則氣散亂。

3. The verb "image" used here means to mentally create something that you treat as if it were real. If you "image" pushing something heavy, you have to adjust your posture exactly as if you were in fact pushing something heavy. You must "feel" its weight, the resistance as you exert force against it, and the force and counterforce in your legs. If you mentally treat your actions as real, your body will too, and the qi will automatically move appropriately for those actions. If you only "pretend" or "imagine" that you are pushing something heavy, your mind and body will not treat your actions as real, and the qi will not move strongly or clearly.

4. 李清菴曰：“調息要調無息息。”

5. 廣成子曰：“一呼則地氣上升，一吸則天氣下降，人之反覆呼吸於蒂，則我之真氣自然相接。”

6. 唱道真言曰：“一呼一吸通乎氣機，一動一靜同乎造化。”

7. 黃庭經曰：“呼吸元氣以求仙。”

8. 伍真人曰：“用後天之呼吸，尋真人呼吸處。”

9. 靈源大道歌：“元和內運即成真，呼吸外求終未了。”

10. 大道教人先止念，念頭不住亦徒然。

11. 無念之念。

12. 孔子曰：“先靜爾后有定，定爾后能安，安爾后能慮，慮爾后能得。”

# Chapter 3. Sitting Eight Pieces of Brocade

It has been nearly one thousand years since the Eight Pieces of Brocade were created. There are many versions, each one somewhat different from the others. However, it does not matter which version you are training, the basic principles and theory are the same, and the goal is consistent. Remember that the most important thing in the training is not the forms themselves, but rather the theory and principle of each form, which constitute the root. Once you understand these, you will be able to use your wisdom mind (yi, 意) to lead the qi to circulate and bring you to health. Therefore, when you practice you should try to understand the poetry or the "secret words." They have been passed down for hundreds of years and are the root of the practice. Because of cultural and language differences, it is very difficult to translate into English all of the meaning of the Chinese. We will try to keep as close as possible to the Chinese and hope that you are able to get not just the meaning, but also the taste of the original. Sometimes, words that are not in the original will be added in parentheses to clarify the meaning. Each section of poetry will be discussed so that it is as clear as possible.

As the first chapter explains, The Eight Pieces of Brocade is an external elixir (wai dan, 外丹) exercise. It includes both types of wai dan qigong practice theory: not only does it build up qi in the limbs and then allow this qi to flow into the organs, but it also uses the motion of the limbs to move the muscles around the organs and increase the qi circulation there.

There are two sets of The Eight Pieces of Brocade. One set is sitting and the other is standing. The sitting set discussed in this chapter focuses on exercising the upper limbs and benefits the six organs that are related to the six qi channels in the arms. The sitting set is a good way to wake up in the morning, and it is usually practiced before noon. The sitting set is also good for people who are bedridden or cannot stand easily.

You may wonder about the number of repetitions given for the different exercises. Chinese people consider twelve to be the number of a cycle; for example, twelve months comprise a year. Therefore, you will often see twelve or its multiples listed as the recommended numbers of repetitions. Square numbers such as nine, sixteen, forty-nine, or sixty-four are also popular. Such numbers are only a guide, and you don't need to follow them precisely. If you have only a limited amount of time and cannot do the recommended number of repetitions, simply use a smaller number. Do not, however, omit any of the exercises.

You may have noticed that in the discussion of the training theory and in the training instructions there is very little about coordinating your breathing with the movements. This is simply because the set was designed for the beginning qigong practitioner. For the beginner, the most important element of the practice is relaxation. Only when you have mastered the set and learned how to regulate your body should you start to coordinate your breath with the movements. The general rule in breathing is that when you extend your limbs you exhale and lead the qi to the extremities, and when you withdraw your limbs you inhale and lead the qi to your spine.

## First Piece

### Close Eyes and Sit Still (Bi Mu Jing Zuo, 閉目靜坐)

閉目冥心坐，握固靜思神。

Translation: Close eyes and sit with deep mind; (hands) hold firm; (mind is) calm, and think (concentrate on the) spirit (shen).

**Practice**

Your mouth is closed and the teeth are touching slightly. Regulate your breathing so that it is smooth and uniform. Your mind is clear and pure. Condense your wisdom mind (yi, 意) and spirit (shen, 神) internally, until the shen is peaceful and the qi sinks. Your

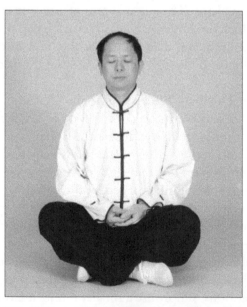

Sit with your legs crossed and concentrate on your solar plexus. Your head should feel as if it were suspended, and your chest loose and relaxed. The waist and spine are easy and comfortable. Hold your hands in your lap.

yi should be at the middle dan tian (solar plexus) first to feel the qi there, then lead the qi down to the lower dan tian (*xia dan tian*, 下丹田). Too much fire qi at middle dan tian is not healthy; it can trigger the heart on fire. Through deep breathing, bring the accumulated fire qi at the middle dan tian to the lower dan tian. You should meditate at least three to five minutes.

**Discussion**

Three places are called fields of elixir (*dan tian*, 丹田): the forehead is called the upper dan tian (*shang dan tian*, 上丹田), the solar plexus is the middle dan tian (*zhong dan tian*, 中丹田), and the abdomen is the lower dan tian (xia dan tian, 下丹田). The upper dan tian is the residence of shen (spirit). When the qi is led to the upper dan tian, the brain is nourished and the spirit can be raised. When the spirit is raised, the qi circulating in the body can be effectively led by the mind. The middle dan tian is the center where the post-birth qi accumulates. Post-birth qi is obtained mainly from food and air. When qi in the middle dan tian is stimulated and full, the body is energized. The mind, however, although stimulated to a higher state, is scattered, and you will be troubled by heartburn. The lower dan tian, which is the original source of human life, is the residence of pre-birth qi.

This exercise will extinguish any fire in your middle dan tian so that you can concentrate and calm your mind. Before you start any qigong exercise, you must first be calm. Closing your eyes will keep you from seeing anything distracting which is happening around you, and help you to calm down. You must train yourself to meditate with a deep mind. When you practice, hold your hands in front of your abdomen. Holding them together will help you to keep your mind centered and firm. If you wish, you may regulate your breath for a minute to start calming your mind, but then let go of the regulating and allow your mind to be calm and deep. You should pay attention to the condition of the post-birth fire qi (hou tian qi, 後天氣) at the middle dan tian, and then lead it down to the lower dan tian to remove excess qi accumulated at the middle dan tian. When the fire is gone, place your concentrated mind on your shen, which is located in the upper dan tian, to increase your energy level.

In China, concentration is called gathering your jing to meet your shen (*ju jing hui shen*, 聚精會神), which implies concentration. Jing here does not mean semen or sperm, but rather something that is refined. Here it means the refined and concentrated mind. When the mind meets with shen (spirit), the shen will be raised. Whenever your shen is raised, you will be able to increase the depth of your concentration.

## Second Piece

### Hands Hold Head (Shou Bao Kun Lun, 手抱崑崙)

扣齒三十六，兩手抱崑崙。

Translation: Knock the teeth thirty-six (times) and two hands hold *kun lun* (head).

**Practice**

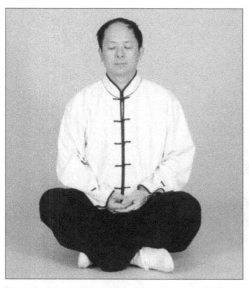

First, tap your teeth together thirty-six times. If there is any saliva generated, swallow it.

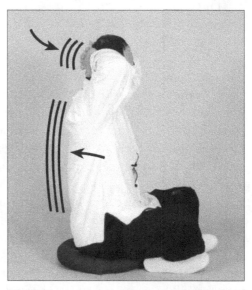

Next, fold your hands together and hold the back of your head. Push your head and body backward while pulling your hands forward. Inhale when tensing and exhale when relaxing. Do nine repetitions.

**Discussion**

There are two major purposes for tapping the teeth together. One purpose is to stimulate the qi in the gums to strengthen the roots of the teeth. In ancient times, dentists and technology were not as common or advanced as today, and you had to take care of your teeth by yourself. Tapping your teeth together strengthens the roots and helps prevent decay. The other purpose is to clear and wake the mind. When you tap, the vibrations resonate in your brain cavity and stimulate the brain. This will clear the mind.

Kun Lun Mountain (崑崙山) is one of the highest mountains in Xinjiang Province (新疆省), China. Here it means your head, which is the highest part of your body. When you push your head backward while pulling your hands forward, also push out your whole back. This will straighten the spine. In addition, this exercise tenses and then relaxes the back muscles, which will increase the qi circulation there and in the governing vessel (du mai, 督脈). This exercise will also strengthen the spine and prevent backache. When you are doing this piece, your breathing should be coordinated with the movement to help the lungs compress and expand. This will release tension in the lungs and increase lung capacity.

## Third Piece

### Knock and Beat the Jade Pillow (Kou Ji Yu Zhen, 叩擊玉枕)

左右鳴天鼓，二十四度聞。

Translation: Left right beat the heavenly drum, resounding twenty-four times.

**Practice**

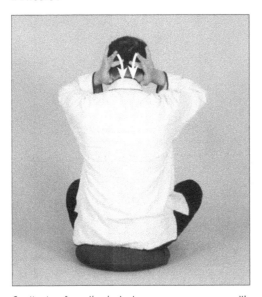

Continuing from the last piece, cover your ears with your palms, with the middle fingers on the jade pillow cavity area (under the external occipital protuberance).

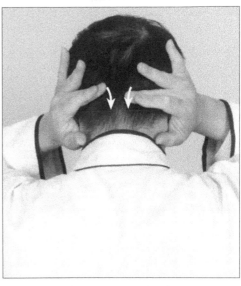

Put your index fingers on the middle fingers and snap them down to hit your head. Hit twenty-four times in an even, steady beat.

This will generate a drumming sound in the brain cavity. This exercise is commonly called "*ming tian gu*" (鳴天鼓) which means "sound the heavenly drum." You may hit with both fingers at the same time, or else alternate the fingers.

**Discussion**

The jade pillow (*yu zhen*, 玉枕) is the name of a cavity located on the back of your head under the protruding ridge of bone. The heavenly drum means the head.

When you do this exercise, do not let your ring and pinkie fingers touch your head, for this will muffle the sound. Concentrate on the sound, and let every beat bring your attention more fully to the vibrations in your skull and brain. Beating the drum clears the mind. When you are finished and take your hands off your ears, you will feel like you just woke up, and everything will seem clear.

## Fourth Piece

### Turn the Head Repeatedly or Lightly Swing the Sky Post (Zhuan Tou Pin Pin or Wei Bai Tian Zhu, 轉頭頻頻 or 微擺天柱)

微擺撼天柱，赤龍攪水津，鼓漱三十六，津液滿口生，一口分三咽，以意送臍輪。

Translation: Lightly turn (the head) to loosen up the *tian zhu* (sky post, i.e. neck). Red dragon (the tongue) stirs the liquid saliva; drum rinse thirty-six (times); saliva liquid fills the entire mouth, one mouthful divided into three swallows, and then use yi to send (it) to the belly wheel (navel).

## Practice

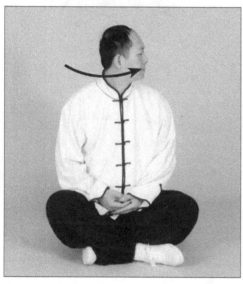

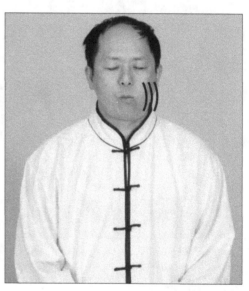

Continuing from the last piece, move your hands down and place them in your lap, palms facing up comfortably. Keeping your shoulders still, turn your head to the left and then the right twenty-four times.

Next, move your tongue around inside your mouth to generate saliva, and then move the saliva around to rinse your mouth thirty-six times, which will also generate more saliva. Swallow this saliva in three gulps. Every time you swallow, use your yi to send the saliva down to the navel.

## Discussion

The head is considered the heavens, and the top of the head is called heavenly cover (*tian ling gai*, 天靈蓋). The neck, which is supported by the two major muscles on the back of the neck, is thus called the tian zhu (天柱), which means the post that supports the heavens. The Chinese word translated here as "loosen up" has the feeling of shaking something to let everything settle back into place. Eight of the fourteen qi channels pass through the neck. As you turn your head back and forth, the neck muscles alternately stretch and relax, which clears the qi channels as well as loosens up the muscles. This prevents the headache caused by stagnation of qi in the head.

According to the Daoists, saliva is the water that is able to put out the fire in the body. For example, when you have a sore throat or heartburn, saliva will ease the pain and help you recover. Saliva is a natural product that is being constantly generated, and it will help you whenever it is needed. When the supply of saliva stops, it is a sign that your body is too positive, and you are about to become ill.

The red dragon refers to the tongue. Move your tongue around in your mouth to generate saliva and then move the saliva around, pushing the cheeks out tight like a drum (drum rinse) to rinse your mouth. Swallowing the saliva will help to put out the fire of excess energy in the heart.

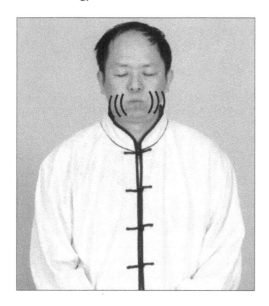

When you swallow, use your mind to lead the saliva down to the lower abdomen. Of course, the saliva doesn't really go that far, but if you act as if you were swallowing the saliva all the way down to your abdomen, you should be able to feel the energy from the saliva sinking to your lower dan tian.

The "belly wheel" or (*qi lun,* 臍輪) is a term the Daoists commonly use for the navel. The Daoists, like the Buddhists, believe that people die and are reborn repeatedly in cycles that move like a great wheel. The abdomen, specifically the navel area, is strongly involved in this reincarnation.

When the text says to bring the saliva to the belly wheel, it actually means the lower dan tian. The Eight Pieces of Brocade is a very simple qigong set, which was designed for the common people. These people would have little or no knowledge of internal things and would not know what the lower dan tian is. The clearest and easiest way was to simply tell them to concentrate on the belly button. Everybody knows where that is, and it is close enough to the lower dan tian to be effective.

## Fifth Piece

### Push and Massage Shenshu or Hands Massage the Essence Door (Tui Mo Shenshu or Shou Mo Jingmen, 推摩腎俞 or 手摩精門)

閉氣搓手熱，背摩後精門，盡此一口氣，想火燒臍輪。

Translation: Seal the breath and rub hands (until) hot, massage the rear essence door (on your) back, end this one mouthful of breath, think (image) the fire is burning the belly wheel.

**Practice**

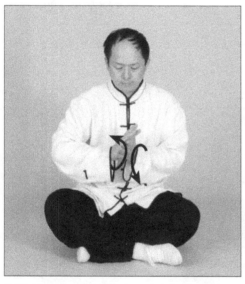

Continuing from the last piece, inhale through your nose and lead the air to the middle dan tian (solar plexus) and hold the breath gently. Rub your hands together until they are warm.

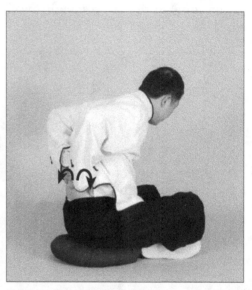

Next, place your palms on the shenshu cavity (B-23, 腎俞) (kidney affirmative) and press in as you massage with a circular motion, twenty-four times.

If you cannot hold your breath comfortably while you massage twenty-four times, don't strain. Only massage twelve times, or however many is comfortable for you, and then exhale. Then inhale again, rub your hands, and repeat. When you massage, unite your yi and qi, and concentrate your yi on the navel or lower dan tian. This concentration will make the abdomen get warm, or even hot. When you are finished with the massaging, sit quietly with your hands in your lap and feel the energy from your kidneys burning inside your navel or lower dan tian.

**Discussion**

Shenshu (B-23, 腎俞) (kidney affirmative), which is also called essence door (*jingmen*, 精門), is the name of a cavity located in the kidney area. There are two of these cavities, one over each kidney. The kidneys are considered the residence of original jing (yuan jing, 元精), also called pre-birth jing. When this jing is converted into qi, it is called original qi (yuan qi, 元氣), and it resides in the lower dan tian (xia dan tian, 下丹田). It is believed that the "essence door" cavities are the doors through which external qi can reach the kidneys, and also the way by which the original qi generated by the kidneys can pass out of the body and be lost. It is also believed that the two kidneys are the roots of the gonads (testicles or ovaries), which the Chinese call the external kidneys. When a person's kidneys are weak, his gonads will function poorly, and hormone production will be deficient. Such a person will be weak, his sexual vitality will be low, and his body will degenerate rapidly.

The person who practices Chinese meditation must learn how to keep from losing his jing through his "essence doors." This is done through lower dan tian breathing, which takes jing from the kidneys and converts it to qi, and stores this qi in the qi residence (lower dan tian, xia dan tian). Therefore, instead of losing your jing, you gain qi, and store it at the lower dan tian.

You must also learn how to use external qi to warm the kidneys and stimulate the production of original qi or jing qi, and how to store it in the lower dan tian so you can use it to improve your health. Therefore, in this piece, you first rub your hands together to generate heat and qi in your hands. When you rub your back with your warm hands, you pass qi into the kidneys, which stimulates them to produce original qi. You don't want this qi to pass out through the "essence doors" and disperse, so you bring it to the lower dan tian. This is done very simply by keeping your attention (yi) on your lower dan tian. Since qi follows yi, the qi you generate will automatically move where you are concentrating. It is said that the more original qi you have stored, the healthier and stronger you will be.

## Sixth Piece

### Hands Turn Double Wheel or Left and Right Windlass (Shou Zhuan Shuang Lun or Zuo You Lu Lu, 手轉雙輪 or 左右轆轤)

手轉雙輪，左右轆轤

Translation: Left and right windlasses turn; two feet lie comfortably extended.

**Practice**

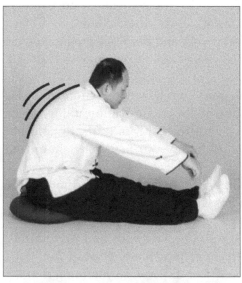

Continuing from the last piece, extend your legs comfortably flat on the floor, with your arms at your sides. Bend forward and extend your arms with palms facing down and the fingers comfortably curved inward.

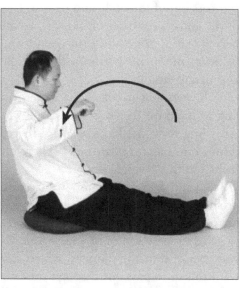

Next, circle your hands upward and backward while slightly bending your upper body backward as if you were rowing a boat.

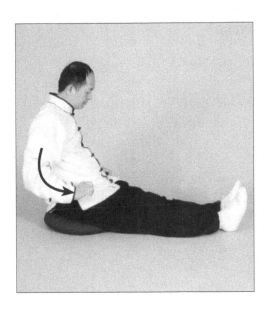

Continue the rowing motion and circle your hands downward and then forward all the way to your feet, to complete the circle. Perform the entire circular motion nine times. Then reverse the direction and repeat the entire circular motion another nine times.

### Discussion

The motion is like turning wheels with both hands. *Lu lu* means turning a wheel or rotating a windlass.

This piece is used mainly to increase qi circulation in the six arm channels. You will feel the qi generated from the circular shoulder motion reaching strongly out to the fingertips. Your legs are stretched out on the floor to open wide the other six qi channels in the legs. Even though you are practicing circulating qi in your hands, the qi will also move out to your toes because your body's natural instinct is to balance the qi throughout your body.

## Seventh Piece

### Lift, Press, and Hold the Feet (Tuo An Pan Zu, 托按攀足)

叉手雙虛托，低頭攀足頻。

Translation: Interlock fingers of both (hands) with false lifting, lower the head repeatedly to hold the feet.

### Practice

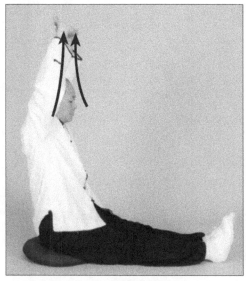

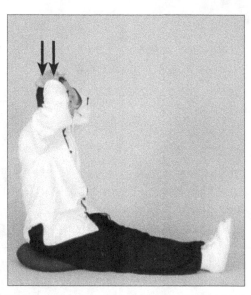

Continuing from the last piece, interlock your hands and lift them above your head, palms up. Keep imaging that you are lifting and holding something up above your head. Stay there for about three seconds. Then turn your palms down and touch the top of your head.

Press your hands downward while you lift your head upward for about three seconds.

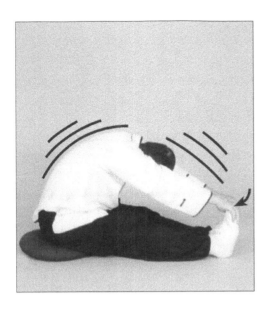

Finally, separate your hands and bend forward, using your hands to pull back your toes. Keep your knees straight and stay in the position for about three seconds. Repeat the entire process nine times.

## Discussion

In this piece, you first interlock your hands and then push up above your head. Because there is nothing for you to push against, the Chinese call it a "false lift." When you push up over your head, you stretch the muscles in the front and back of your body. This stretching and relaxing movement helps to regulate the *sanjiao qi* channels. Sanjiao means "triple burner" and includes the upper, middle, and lower parts of your torso. The upper burner is located in the chest above the diaphragm, the middle burner is between the diaphragm and the navel, and the lower burner is located between the navel and the groin.

After you have loosened up the muscles, place your hands on the top of your head and press down. You balance this downward push with an upward push of your head. This upward push comes all the way from the floor. The yi of pushing upward and downward will lead any stagnant qi in the sanjiao areas into the small circulation (the circular pathway through the conception and governing vessels).

Finally, hold your toes or feet and pull them back, letting your head hang down. This position stretches and slightly tenses the muscles in the back. When you then sit up and raise your arms over your head, you release the tension. This alternately presses in on the kidneys and then lets up, which increases the circulation of blood and qi in the kidneys and keeps them healthy.

Another way to do the last part of this piece is to place your hands over your toes and press your middle fingers into the bubbling well cavities. Since these cavities are on the channels that connect with the kidneys, this method provides additional stimulation to the kidneys.

## Eighth Piece

### Entire Sky Slow Transportation (Zhou Tian Man Yun, 周天慢運)

以候口水至，　再漱再吞津，　如此三度畢，　口水九次吞，
咽下汨汨響，　百脈自調勻，　周天慢運畢，　想火遍燒身。
舊名八段錦，　子後午前行，　勤行無間斷，　萬病化為塵。

Translation: Wait until the mouth water arrives, again rinse, again swallow the saliva; do this three times, swallow mouth water nine times, swallow noisily; (in) hundreds of vessels (qi) adjusts uniformly (and) automatically, and entire sky (body) slow transportation completed; think that fire is burning (your) entire body. Ancient name: Eight Pieces of Brocade; train after midnight and before noon, train diligently without ceasing, thousands of illnesses vanish into dust.

### Practice

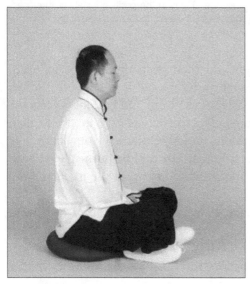

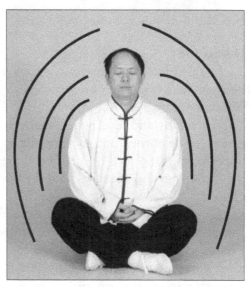

Cross your legs and place your hands in your lap. Close your eyes and sit calmly. When enough saliva accumulates, rinse and then swallow three times with an audible gulp. After you swallow, keep your attention on your navel or lower dan tian, and feel the qi circulating smoothly throughout your body. When more saliva accumulates, rinse again and swallow three more times. Repeat once more, for a total of nine swallows.

Next, relax and feel the qi burning like a fire all over your body. This means that you should lead the qi to your skin to form a protective shield around your body.

### Discussion

When you have finished the preceding seven pieces, your body may be too positive, and you may have let qi rise up in your body instead of settle down to the lower dan tian. Swallowing the saliva is a way to bring the qi back down again. There are two ways to generate saliva. One is to move the tongue around in the mouth, and the other is to simply concentrate your mind on your mouth and let the saliva be generated spontaneously. Since this is the last piece, it is desirable to put out any fire you may have caused by the exercises. If you start moving your tongue around again, you may start generating more heat and fire. You simply want to calm down. That is why you use your yi instead of your tongue to generate the saliva. In this piece, when you swallow, you do it "noisily." Bringing the saliva down with a big gulp helps to concentrate all of your attention and makes it easier for you to relax.

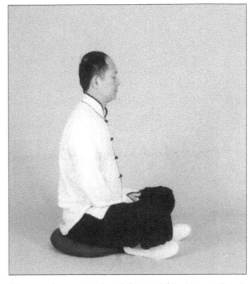

After you have completed these eight pieces, sit quietly and breathe evenly for about three minutes.

You want the qi you have accumulated in your lower dan tian to circulate throughout your body. When you sit quietly with your attention on your lower dan tian, the qi will accumulate there. As it fills up the lower dan tian, it will become stimulated, gradually spreading out and filling the entire body. You will be able to feel the qi moving throughout your body, clearing out obstructions in the channels and automatically balancing itself. You may feel the qi moving through what is called the small circulation (*xiao zhou tian*, 小周天), which is the circular path through the governing vessel (up) on the back of the torso and then through the conception vessel (down) the center front of the torso.

When you are finished with the swallowing and the body is warm and full of qi, imagine that the skin and the area around your body is full of fire. This image will bring qi to the skin and build up the shield of guardian qi (wei qi, 衛氣) around the body.

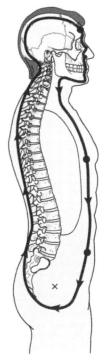

Small circulation.

# Chapter 4. Standing Eight Pieces of Brocade

The standing set of the Eight Pieces of Brocade is more popular than the sitting set, so there are more versions of it in the documents. You should not worry about which version is better or more accurate because the basic principles are the same. It is more important that you really understand the root of the practice and that you train patiently and perseveringly. Every piece has its own poem or song to explain the exercise and its purpose. The poems or songs have been passed down through generations and form the root and foundation of each piece, so you should make a diligent effort to understand them. Whereas the sitting set emphasized the six qi channels in the arms, the standing set works with all of the channels.

## First Piece

### Double Hands Hold up the Heavens

雙手托天理三焦，三焦通暢疾病消。
反手朝天振雙臂，挺胸直腰兩側搖。
立正姿勢要站穩，久練體壯樂陶陶。

Translation: Double hands hold up the heavens to regulate the triple burner (sanjiao, 三焦); sanjiao passes (qi) freely and smoothly, illnesses disappear. Reverse hands to face the sky and raise both arms. Thrust out (straighten) your chest; straighten your waist (and) swing to both sides. Stand upright and be steady. Practice long; the body (becomes) strong (and you will feel) happy.

### Practice

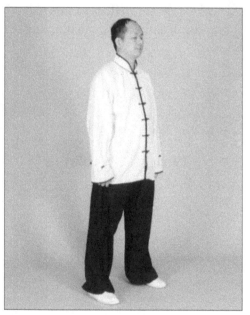

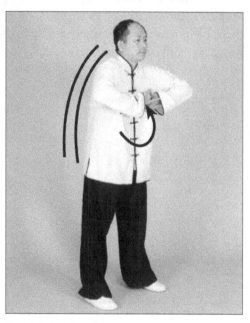

Stand naturally with your feet parallel and shoulder width apart, and your hands at your sides. Close your eyes, calm down your mind, and breathe regularly. Open your eyes and look forward, continue breathing naturally and smoothly.

Next, interlock your fingers.

Condense your spirit (shen, 神) in your upper dan tian, and sink your qi to the lower dan tian (xia dan tian, 下丹田).

This is called "double hands hold up the heavens" (*shuang shou tuo tian*, 雙手托天).

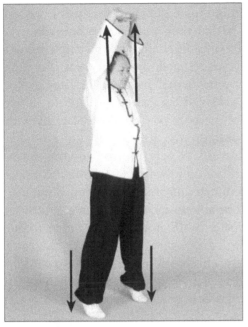

Raise your hands above your head without bending your arms, and at the same time lift up your heels.

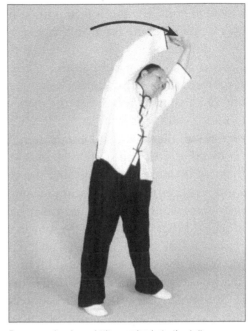

Drop your heels and tilt your body to the left.

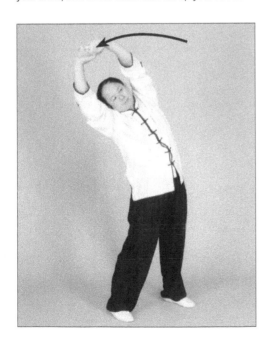

Next, tilt your body to the right, and then stand up straight again, keeping your hands over your head.

Then gently lower your hands down in front of your body and stand naturally to complete one round. Your feet should be parallel and shoulder width apart, and your hands at your sides. Repeat the entire process twenty-four times.

## Discussion

This set does not start with calm meditation, but since qigong training is strongly related to your feelings, it is important for your mind to be calm and steady. It is a good idea to stand quietly for a while before you start so that your mind can become calm.

From the poetry, you can see that this piece works especially with the triple burner (sanjiao, 三焦). The three areas, or "burners" that are referred to, are the areas above the diaphragm: The upper burner is between the diaphragm and navel (shang jiao, 上焦); the middle burner is between the navel and the groin (zhong jiao, 中焦); and the lower burner is called the (xia jiao, 下焦). The three burners are concerned respectively with respiration, digestion, and elimination. When you raise your hands over your head and tilt to either side, you stretch the muscles of your trunk. When you let your arms down, the muscles loosen and relax, and the qi can circulate unimpeded. Repeating the movement regulates the qi circulation in your sanjiao. When sanjiao qi circulation is smooth, the organs will be relaxed, and the organ qi will be able to move and circulate freely. It is believed that disorders in the sanjiao are the major cause of many qi disorders to our organs. When sanjiao qi is regulated, the illness will disappear.

When you practice, you also lift up your heels. This helps you to generate a wisdom mind (yi, 意) of pushing up, which helps the sanjiao qi move up and down. When we say to "straighten your waist," we mean to keep your lower back straight.

## Second Piece

### Left Right Open the Bow

左右開弓似射雕，兩臂堅牢壯腎腰。
曲肘平肩努力拉，手箭對準用目瞄。
左右放射二十四，騎馬蹲襠效力高。

Translation: Left right open (bend) the bow, like shooting a hawk, your two arms strong and firm to strengthen kidneys and waist. Bend the elbow horizontal to the shoulder, (your mind) trying hard to pull. Arrow in hands aims (at the target) and uses the eyes to stare. Left right shoot for twenty-four times. Ride the horse and squat down to increase efficiency.

### Practice

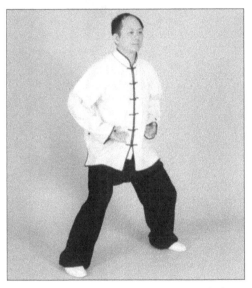

From a natural standing position, step your right leg to the right and squat down in a horse stance.

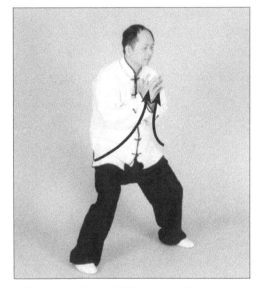

Relax your hands and lift them up to the chest area. Bring your palms together.

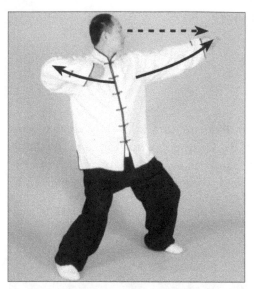

Next, separate your hands with your right hand moving near your right nipple, while your left hand, changing into the "sword secret" (*jian jue*, 劍訣) or "single finger" (*yi zhi chan*, 一指禪) hand form, extends outward to the left. The motion is as if you were pulling a bowstring to shoot a hawk. Your eyes stare to your left at a very distant point.

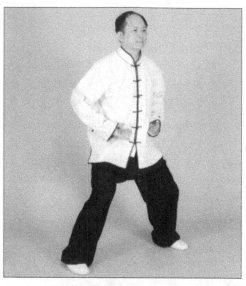

Raise your body slightly, and simultaneously lower your hands. Then squat down in a horse stance.

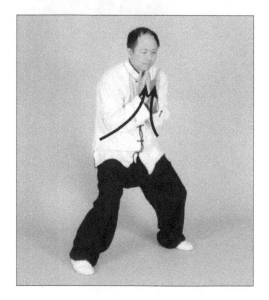

Relax your hands and lift them up to the chest area. Bring your palms together.

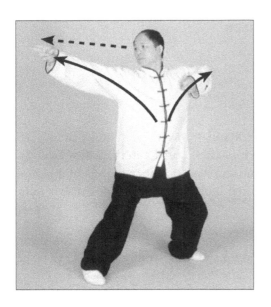

Next, separate your hands with the left hand moving near the left nipple, while the right hand, changing into the "sword secret" (jian jue, 劍訣) or "single finger" (yi zhi chan, 一指禪) hand form, extends outward to the right. Do twelve in each direction for a total of twenty-four repetitions.

## Discussion

This piece is used to strengthen the kidneys and the waist area. First, you must squat down to firm your root as when you pull a strong bow. Without this root, you will not have a center, and you will not be able to pull your bow effectively. Make sure when you squat down that you keep your back straight and tuck your buttocks under. This emphasizes the kidney area. When you are doing this, you not only strengthen the waist muscles but also increase the qi circulation in the kidney area in your back near your lowest ribs. Your rear elbow must be bent and the shoulders must be firm to stabilize the pulling of the bow. Concentrate your mind so that you actually feel that you are drawing a very strong bow. This concentrated mind is the source of the qi movement.

## Third Piece

### Lift Singly

調理脾胃須單舉，脾胃平和病自癒。
舉臂挺掌用力搖，伸撥筋肋脾胃舒。
右手高舉左下垂，左右伸搖筋絡活。

Translation: To adjust and regulate the spleen and stomach (you) must lift singly; spleen and stomach (to gain) peace and harmony; sickness cured automatically. Lift arm and stiffen the palms, use the force to rock. Extend and develop the tendons and muscles, spleen and stomach comfortably. Right hand lifted high, left dropped down, left right extend, and rock the tendons and channels alive.

### Practice

After you have completed the last piece, stand up and move your leg back so that the feet are parallel and shoulder width apart.

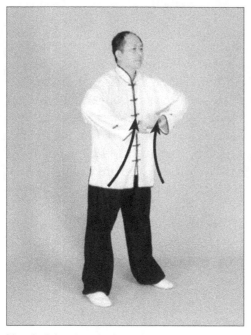

Move both hands to the front of your stomach with the palms facing up.

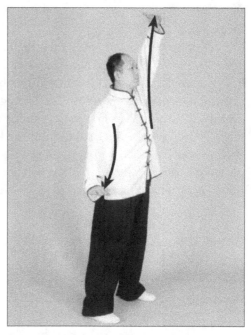

Raise your left hand above your head and push upward, and at the same time lower your right hand palm down to your side and press down slightly.

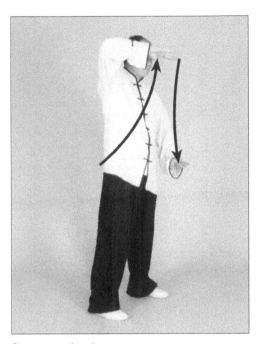

Change your hands.

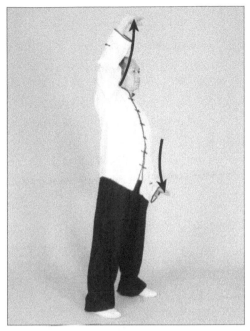

Raise your right hand above your head and push upward, and at the same time lower your left hand palm down to your side and press down slightly. You should feel that both hands are pushing against resistance, but you must not tense your muscles. Do twelve on each side for a total of twenty-four repetitions.

## Discussion

This piece works on the stomach. When you repeatedly raise one hand and lower the other, you loosen the muscles in the front of your body. When you "stiffen the palms," do not tense the muscles, but rather extend your force through the hands so that your arms stretch out all the way. This stimulates and strengthens the tendons and muscles. Reversing your arms repeatedly stretches and relaxes the body, "rocking" the tendons and qi channels alive. This one-up-and-one-down muscle movement increases the qi circulation in your stomach, spleen, and liver. If you wish, when you raise and stretch each hand you can also stretch the leg on the same side to increase the extension.

## Fourth Piece

### Five Weaknesses and Seven Injuries

五勞七傷望後瞧，久練久作筋骨牢。
勞傷皆因內臟弱，挺胸扭脖後看好。
搯腰捧胸身平立，專治內傷有功效。

Translation: Five weaknesses and seven injuries—wait and see later (they'll be gone); train long, exercise long, tendons and bones strong. Weakness injuries (from over-exertion) all because the internal organs (are) weak. Thrust out (straighten) the chest and twist the neck to take a good look to the rear. Hold the waist and hold up the chest; the body is upright. This is especially effective in curing internal injury.

### Practice

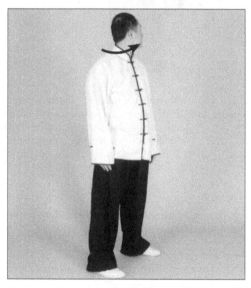

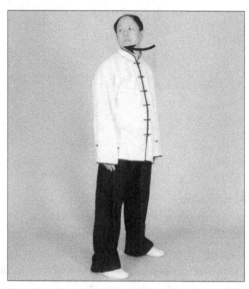

Stand easily and comfortably with both feet parallel, and your hands hanging down naturally at your sides. Lift your chest slightly from the inside so that your posture is straight, but be careful not to thrust your chest out. Turn your head to the left and look to the rear as you exhale.

Next, return your head to the front as you inhale. Turn your head to the right and look to the rear as you exhale. Return your head to the front as you inhale. Turn twelve times in each direction, for a total of twenty-four. Your body should remain facing to the front. Do not turn your body as you turn your head.

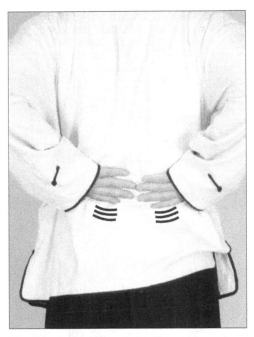

Place your hands on your waist. Thumbs forward and fingertips point to your spine.

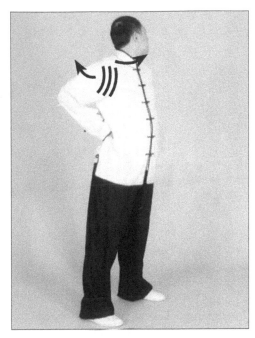

Turn your head to the left and look to the rear as you exhale.

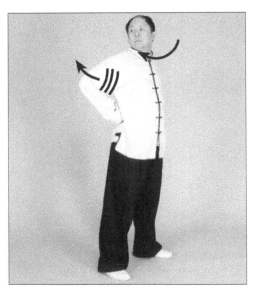

Return your head to the front as you inhale. Turn your head to the right and look to the rear as you exhale. Return your head to the front as you inhale. Turn twelve times in each direction, for a total of twenty-four. Your body should remain facing to the front. Do not turn your body as you turn your head.

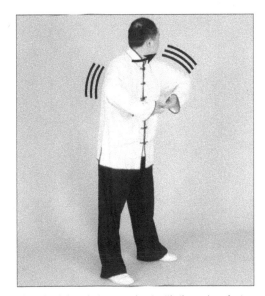

Move both hands to your chest with the palms facing up, press your elbows and shoulders slightly forward, and turn your head to the left as you exhale.

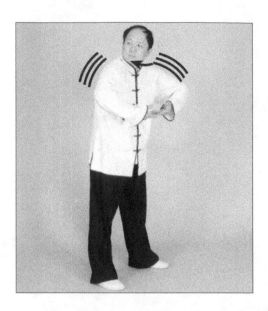

Return your head to the front as you inhale. Turn your head to the right as you exhale. Return your head to the front as you inhale. Turn twelve times in each direction, for a total of twenty-four. Your body should remain facing to the front. Do not turn your body as you turn your head.

During all three parts, use your yi to lead the qi from the lower dan tian to your bubbling well (yongquan, K-1) and huiyin cavities when you exhale and turn your head to either side, and then lead the qi back to the lower dan tian as you inhale and return your head to the front.

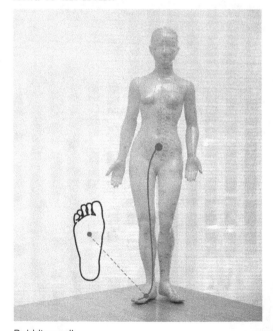

Bubbling well.

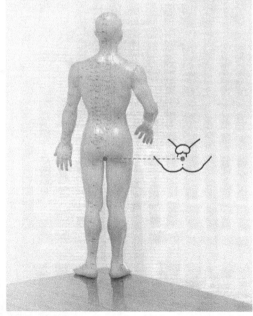

Huiyin cavity.

**Discussion**

Five weaknesses (五勞) refer to illnesses of the five yin organs: heart, liver, spleen, lungs, and kidneys. The seven injuries (七傷) refer to injuries caused by the seven emotions: happiness, anger, sorrow, joy, love, hate, and desire. According to Chinese medicine, you can become ill when your internal organs are weak and emotional disturbance upsets them. For example, anger can cause the qi in your liver to stagnate, which will affect the functioning of the organ. But your organs are not the only things affected—strong emotions also cause qi to accumulate in your head. When you turn your head from side to side you loosen up the muscles, blood vessels, and qi channels in your neck and allow the qi in your head to smooth out. Additionally, since you are also training your feelings and shen to be centered and neutral, you will be able to avoid excessive or extreme emotions and their negative effects. In the form, you turn your head to look behind you, as if you were looking at all the negative things that you have left behind. It is important to look intently to the rear, so that the qi keeps moving. If you merely turn your head, the qi will stagnate in your neck. Practicing this piece regularly will regulate the qi in your organs and head, repairing the damage caused by strong emotions and helping you to avoid all illnesses.

The poem also implies that this piece can cure old injuries. When you practice, you use your mind to lead the qi from your lower dan tian to the bubbling well cavities, which smoothes out the qi circulation in your lower body. When you turn your head while holding your hands in the different positions, you slightly stretch different parts of the inside of your body and regulate the qi flow there. This will help to cure old internal injuries and bruises that cannot be easily reached by other methods of treatment.

## Fifth Piece

### Sway the Head and Swing the Tail to get rid of the Heart Fire

頭擺尾去心火，心火旺盛肺金克。
手按膝蓋多搖擺，血液暢流好處多。
筋攣腿酸身麻木，重伸重壓莫蹉跎。

Translation: Sway the head and swing the tail to get rid of the heart fire. (When) the heart fire (is) strong, (use) the metal lung to subdue. Hands press the kneecaps, repeatedly sway and swing. Blood flows smoothly, many good benefits. (If) the muscles/tendons are cramped, legs sore, (and) body numb, repeatedly extend and press heavily; do not waste time (hesitate).

### Practice

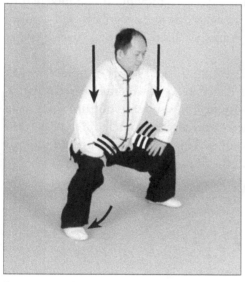

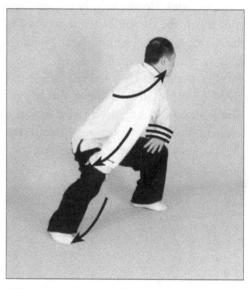

From a natural standing position, step your right leg one step to the right and squat down in a horse stance. Place your hands on top of your knees, with the thumbs on the outside of the thighs. Your qi is sunk to the bottom of your feet, and your yi is on the two bubbling well cavities.

Shift your weight to your left leg and press down heavily with your hand, and line up (extend) your head, spine, and right leg. Stay in this position for about three seconds.

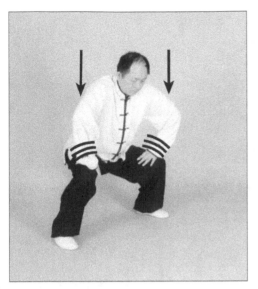

Return to the original position.

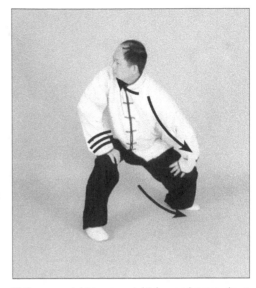

Shift your weight to your right leg and press down heavily with your hand, and line up (extend) your head, spine, and right leg. Stay in this position for about three seconds. Turn twelve times in each direction for a total of twenty-four repetitions.

## Discussion

Fire (excessive qi) in the middle dan tian (zhong dan tian, 中丹田) at the solar plexus can be caused by improper food, breathing unhealthy air, or lack of sleep. This frequently causes heartburn. For this reason, it is called heart fire (*xin huo*, 心火). When excessive qi accumulates and stagnates in your middle dan tian or heart, the best course of action is to move this fire to the lungs where you can regulate it and put it out with smooth breathing. According to the five elements theory, fire can destroy metal, but metal can also absorb the heat and control fire. The lungs belong to the element metal (Table 1), and the heart belongs to the element fire, and so it is said that the metal lungs can subdue the heart fire. When you hold your hands on your knees with the thumbs to the rear, you are expanding your chest, and when you move your body from side to side, you are loosening up the lungs and therefore taking in the excess qi from the middle dan tian, and consequently putting out the fire. As you are doing this, you are also increasing the blood circulation, which will take care of any numbness or soreness in the legs.

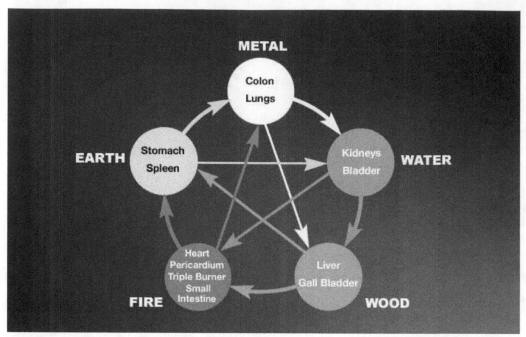

Five elements.

| | WOOD 木 | FIRE 火 | EARTH 土 | METAL 金 | WATER 水 |
|---|---|---|---|---|---|
| Direction | East | South | Center | West | North |
| Season | Spring | Summer | Long Summer | Autumn | Winter |
| Climactic Condition | Wind | Summer Heat | Dampness | Dryness | Cold |
| Process | Birth | Growth | Transformation | Harvest | Storage |
| Color | Green | Red | Yellow | White | Black |
| Taste | Sour | Bitter | Sweet | Pungent | Salty |
| Smell | Goatish | Burning | Fragrant | Rank | Rotten |
| Yin Organ | Liver | Heart | Spleen | Lungs | Kidneys |
| Yang Organ | Gall Bladder | Small Intestine | Stomach | Large Intestine | Bladder |
| Opening | Eyes | Tongue | Mouth | Nose | Ears |
| Tissue | Sinews | Blood Vessels | Flesh | Skin/Hair | Bones |
| Emotion | Anger | Happiness | Pensiveness | Sadness | Fear |
| Human Sound | Shout | Laughter | Song | Weeping | Groan |

Table 1. Table of the Five Basic Elements showing their impact on human life.

Make sure that when you lean to each side you don't drop your head. Keep your head, neck, and spine in a line. When you "press heavily" on one knee, you compress the lung on that side and relax and open the lung on the other side. This works the two lungs like bellows.

## Sixth Piece

### Two Hands Hold the Feet

雙手攀足固腎腰，腎腰充實整體牢。
腎身彎腰手攀足，強筋壯骨有功效。
一落一起活力大，防止感冒更為佳。

Translation: Two hands hold the feet to strengthen the kidneys and waist; (when the) kidneys and waist are strong the entire body (is) strong. Bend the waist and hold the feet. (This is the) most effective way to strengthen the muscles/tendons and bones. One down one up, the life force greatly increases. (It is) the best way to prevent colds.

### Practice

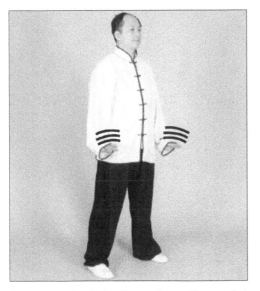

Assume a natural standing posture with your feet shoulder-width apart. Press both palms down slightly beside your waist.

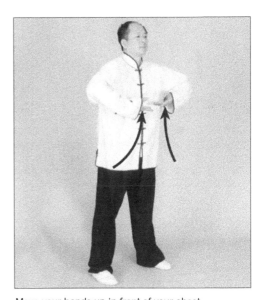

Move your hands up in front of your chest.

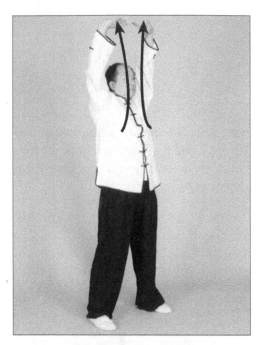

Continue to move your hands above your head with the palms facing up. Hold the posture for three seconds. The form looks as if you are holding or lifting something above your head. Your mind is on your mingmen cavity (Gv-4, 命門) in the kidney area.

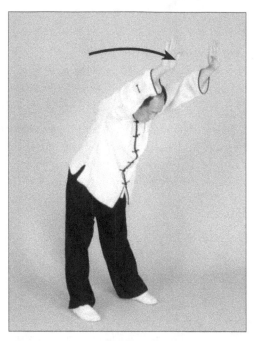

Bend forward with the arms extended.

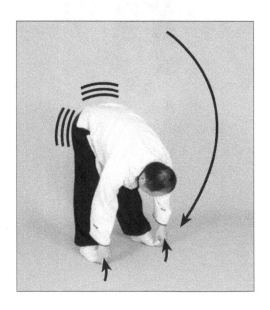

Grab your toes and hold your feet. Pull your hands up slightly so that you are putting a gentle stress on your whole body. While holding your feet, your mind is on the bubbling well (yongquan, K-1, 湧泉) cavity. Hold the posture for three seconds. Perform the entire process sixteen times.

**Discussion**

The kidneys, which are beneath the two major back muscles, are the residence of original jing (yuan jing, 元精). When the kidneys are healthy and strong, your original jing is retained and strengthened. Only when your kidneys are strong will they be able to generate original qi (yuan qi, 元氣) and enliven your body. When you bend forward and use your hands to hold your feet, you are tensing the back muscles and restricting the flow of qi in the area of the kidneys. When you release this pressure, the qi flow will resume, removing any qi stagnation. This exercise is an excellent way to massage the kidneys and increase the flow of qi there, as well as in the back muscles and the spine itself. When the kidneys are strong, the original qi will be strong. When original qi is full and strong, your body will be able to generate a strong shield of guardian qi (wei qi, 衛氣) to protect you from the cold.

When you are bent over you are lightly stressing your whole body, and in particular, you are stimulating your kidneys. When you straighten up and extend your arms, your mind is thinking of stretching out to your hands and feet. This action of the mind and body leads the qi out to all your tendons. When you are bent over, part of your attention (and part of the qi from your kidneys) is drawn to your sacrum. The qi will enter the spine through the holes in the sacrum, and when you stand up it will pass through the spine. Eventually the qi will move through and vitalize your whole skeleton.

## Seventh Piece

### Screw the Fist with Fiery Eyes

攢拳怒目增氣力，身心健康精神爽。
騎馬蹲襠胸挺直，握拳擊掌多用力。
左右兩手循環抓，抓握怒目用力氣。

Translation: Screw the fist with fiery eyes to increase *qi-li*; body and mind healthy, the spirit of vitality comfortable. Ride the horse and squat down, straightening the chest. Hold the fist or strike with palm, using more force. Left and right, two hands grasp in turn. Grasp, hold, fiery eyes, use *li-qi*.

### Practice

This piece is very similar to the second piece.

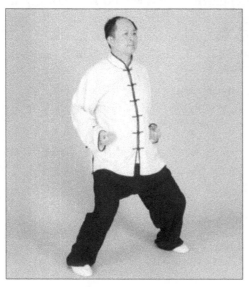 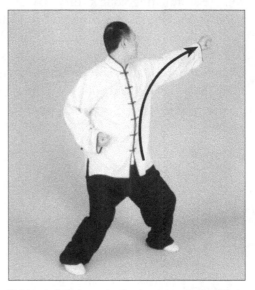

From a natural standing posture, step your right foot to the side and squat down in a horse stance, holding your body erect and your fists beside your waist.

Tighten both fists, and extend one arm to the side in a twisting punch motion (screw the fist). Your other hand stays beside your waist in a tight fist. The hand that is out can be either a fist or an open palm. When you make the punching motion, glare fiercely at an imaginary opponent.

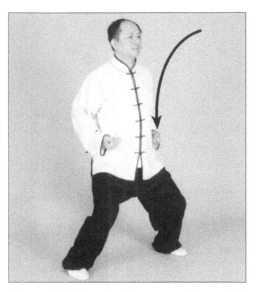

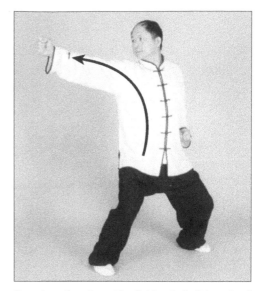

After you finish the extending movement, loosen both hands and bring the extended hand back to your waist to the starting position.

Repeat on the other side. Tighten both fists, extend one arm to the side in a twisting punch motion (screw the fist). Your other hand stays beside your waist in a tight fist. The hand that is out can be either a fist or an open palm. When you make the punching motion, glare fiercely at an imaginary opponent. Do eight on both sides, for a total of sixteen repititions.

## Discussion

This piece trains you to raise your spirit of vitality. When your spirit is raised, you strengthen the qi flow and also increase your muscular strength (*li*, 力). Muscular strength that is reinforced by qi is called qi-li (氣力) or li-qi (力氣). As you raise your spirit (shen, 神) and increase your qi-li, the qi will fill your body all the way out to the skin. In the other exercises, you have been focusing your attention and concentrating your qi. It is important to now do this piece because it clears out any stagnant qi and leads it to the skin. Concentrating your yi is the key to success. If you have a very strong mental image of punching someone very hard, your yi will lead your qi out to the ends of your arms and legs to make the punch powerful.

## Eighth Piece

### Seven Disorders and Hundreds of Illnesses Disappear

背後七顛百病消，百病皆因體弱招。
足顛功能筆難描，頭頂震到腳趾稍。
搖腰捧胸上下顛，卻病消災有功效。

Translation: Seven disorders and hundreds of illnesses disappear and are left behind your back; hundreds of illnesses are caused because the body is weak. The feet up, achievement is hard to describe by pen. Keep the head up and press down to reach to the end of the toes. Hold the waist and hold the chest, up and down movements. (It is) effective in getting rid of sickness and eliminating disasters (illnesses).

### Practice

There are three parts to this exercise. The different hand positions serve different qi circulation functions.

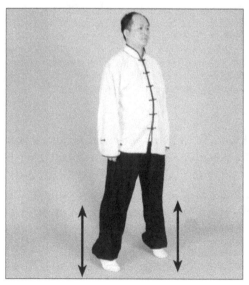

First, drop both hands down naturally, beside your body. Stand still and keep your mind calm. Rise up on your toes and stay as high as you can for three seconds, then lower your feet to the floor. Perform the motion twenty-four times.

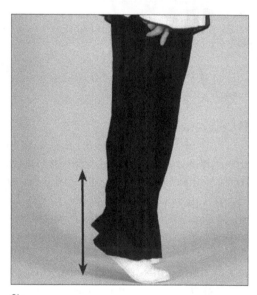

Close-up.

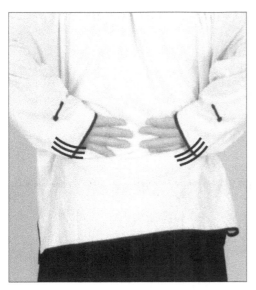

Place your hands on your waist. Thumbs forward and fingertips pointing to your spine.

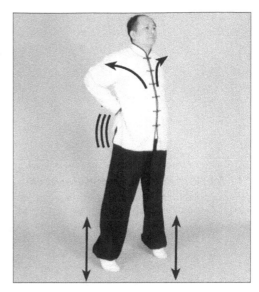

Raise yourself up on your toes for three seconds and then let yourself down. Do this twenty-four times.

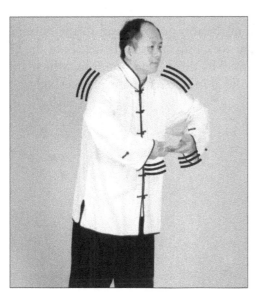

Hold your hands in front of your chest.

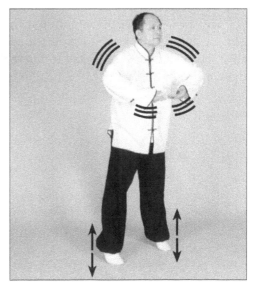

Raise yourself up on your toes for three seconds and then let yourself down. Do this twenty-four times.

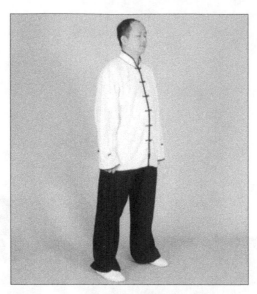

After you finish this piece, stand still, keep your mind calm, and breathe smoothly and regularly for about three minutes.

## Discussion

This piece is used to smooth out the qi from the top of your head to the bottom of your feet. When you raise yourself up on your toes, you are stimulating six of the qi channels, which are connected to internal organs. The three hand positions, which are the same as in the fourth piece, help to regulate the qi in different parts of your body.

# Chapter 5. Conclusion

As mentioned in chapter one, Chinese qigong has a number of different styles, or schools, which come from different sources. One style, which was developed by scholars and is now practiced by the general populace, is devoted to maintaining health. A second style developed by Chinese doctors concentrates on healing. A third style was developed in the Buddhist and Daoist religions to help the devotees reach the goal of immortality. This style seeks not only to improve and maintain health, but also to lengthen life.

Once you become familiar with the Eight Pieces of Brocade, you will find that it is a very simple but effective way to maintain your health. You may also notice that, unlike the sets developed by doctors and monks, breath coordination is not essential in most of the pieces. The Eight Pieces of Brocade follow a few simple principles, but they will lead the interested practitioner down the right path to discover what qi is all about and will also improve health.

I hope this simple set of qigong practice will help you to have a healthy life, and encourage you to get involved in further qigong study and research. If you have obtained benefit from this set, please introduce it to your friends and help them to improve their health.

# Glossary and Chinese Terms

**Ba Duan Jin** (八段錦). Eight Pieces of Brocade, wai dan qigong practice created by Marshal Yue, Fei (岳飛) during the Southern Song dynasty (南宋) (AD 1127–1279).

**bagua** (八卦). Eight divinations, also called the eight trigrams. Shown in the *Yi Jing* as groups of single and broken lines. Also called bakua.

**Baguazhang (Ba Kua Chang)** (八卦掌). Eight Trigrams Palm. One of the internal qigong martial styles believed to have been created by Dong, Hai-chuan, during (AD 1866–1880).

**Bai He** (白鶴). White Crane, one of the Chinese southern martial styles.

**ba kua** (八卦). See **bagua.**

*Bao Pu Zi* (抱朴子). Qigong and Chinese medical book that advocates using the mind to lead and increase Qi. Written during the Jin dynasty in the third century AD. See also **Ge, Hong.**

*Bao Shen Mi Yao* (保身祕要). A qigong and medical book that described moving and stationary qigong practices. See also **Cao, Yuan-bai.**

**Bian Que** (扁鵲). Physician who wrote the book, *Classic on Disorders* (*Nan Jing*, 難經) during Chinese Qin and Han dynasties (秦，漢) (221 BC–AD 220). See also *Nan Jing.*

**bian shi** (砭石). Stone probes used before metal needles were available for acupuncture.

**Cao, Yuan-bai** (曹元白). Physician and qigong master who wrote *The Secret Important Document of Body Protection* (*Bao Shen Mi Yao*, 保身祕要) during the Qing dynasty (清) (AD 1644–1911). See also *Bao Shen Mi Yao.*

**Chan (Ren)** (禪 or 忍) A Chinese school of Mahayana Buddhism, which asserts that enlightenment can be attained through meditation, self-contemplation, and intuition, rather than through study of scripture. Chan (Ren) is commonly known as Zen in Japan.

**chang** (長) Long.

**Chang Chuan** (長拳). See **Changquan.**

**Changquan** (長拳). Includes all northern Chinese long-range martial styles.

**Chang, Xiang-san** (張詳三). A well-known Chinese martial artist in Taiwan.

**Chao, Yuan-fang** (巢元方). Physician and qigong master from the Sui and Tang dynasties who compiled 260 different ways of increasing the qi flow. See also *Zhu Bing Yuan Hou Lun.*

**Chen, Ji-ru** (陳繼儒). Physician and qigong master from Qing dynasty who wrote book about the three treasures: essence, internal energy, and spirit. See also *Yang Sheng Fu Yu.*

**Chen, Wilson** (陳威伸). Dr. Yang, Jwing-Ming's friend.

**Cheng, Gin-gsao** (曾金灶). Dr. Yang, Jwing-Ming's White Crane master.

**chi** (氣). See **qi**.

**chi kung** (氣功) See **qigong**.

**chin na** (擒拿). A component of Chinese martial arts that emphasizes grabbing techniques, to control your opponent's joints, in conjunction with attacking certain acupuncture cavities.

**chong mai** (衝脈). Thrusting vessel. One of the eight extraordinary qi vessels.

**Chun Qiu Zhan Guo** (春秋戰國). Spring and Autumn Warring Periods, in Chinese history, (722–222 BC).

**Da Mo** ( 達摩). The Indian Buddhist monk, also known as Bodhidarma, who is credited with creating the *Yi Jin Jing* and *Xi Sui Jing* while at the Shaolin monastery. Before he was a monk, his last name was Sardili, prince of a small tribe in southern India.

**da zhou tian** (大周天). Translated as grand circulation. After a nei dan qigong (內丹氣功) practitioner completes small circulation (xiao zhou tian, 小周天), he will circulate his qi through the entire body or exchange the qi with nature. See also **xiao zhou tian; nei dan**.

**dan tian** (丹田). Locations in the body that can store and generate qi. The upper, middle, and lower dan tian are located respectively between the eyebrows, at the solar plexus, and a few inches below the navel.

**Dao** (道). The way, by implication, the "natural way."

***Dao De Jing*** (道德經). *Morality Classic* written by Lao Zi (老子).

**Dao Jia** (道家). Daoism, as created by Lao Zi during the Zhou dynasty (周) (1122–934 BC).

**Dao Jiao** (道教). Daoist religion created by Zhang, Dao-ling who combined traditional Daoist principles with Buddhism during the Chinese Han dynasty (漢) (c. AD 58).

**di** (地). The earth, one of the "three natural powers" (san cai, 三才).

**di li shi** (地理師). Di li means "geomancy" and shi means "teacher," a teacher or master who analyzes geographic locations according to the formulas in the *Book of Changes* (*Yi Jing,* 易經) and the energy distributions in the earth. See also **feng shui shi**.

**di qi** (地氣). The energy of the earth.

**Dong Han dynasty** (東漢). A Chinese dynasty, (AD 25–168).

**Dong, Hai-chuan** (董海川). Chinese internal martial artist who is credited with the creation of Baguazhang (八卦掌) in the late Qing dynasty (清) (AD 1644–1911).

**du mai** (督脈). The "governing vessel," one of the eight extraordinary vessels.

**feng shui shi** (風水師). Called a wind, water teacher or master of geomancy, which is the art or science of analyzing the natural energy relationships in a location, especially the interrelationships between "wind" and "water." See also **di li shi**.

**Ge, Hong** (葛洪). Physician and qigong master who wrote the book, *Bao Pu Zi* (抱朴子) during the Jin dynasty (晉), third century AD. See also ***Bao Pu Zi.***

***Ge Zhi Yu Lun*** (格致餘論). *A Further Thesis of Complete Study,* medical and qigong thesis explaining how gigong could cure illness. Written by Zhu, Dan-xi, (宋，金，元) (AD 960–1368). See also **Zhu, Dan-xi.**

**gongfu** (功夫). Means "energy-time." Anything that takes time and energy to learn or to accomplish is called gongfu. Also known as kung fu.

**guai zi ma** (枴子馬). The guai zi ma was an ancient version of the tank. It was a chariot carrying armored men, drawn by three fully armored horses connected by a chain. Guai zi ma was invented by the Jin (金) general Wu Zhu (兀朮) during the Chinese Song dynasty (宋).

**Guang Cheng Zi** (廣成子). A well-known Daoist qigong master who lived from (AD 1140–1212), during the Chinese Jin dynasty (金).

**guoshu** (國術). Combined and abbreviated form of zhongguo and wushu (中國武術), which means "Chinese martial techniques."

**Han dynasty** (漢朝). A dynasty in Chinese history from (206 BC–AD 221).

**Han, Qi** (韓琦). Marshal Yue, Fei's landlord when Fei was a child.

**Han, Ching-tang** (韓慶堂). A well-known Chinese martial artist, especially in Taiwan in the last sixty years. Master Han is also Dr. Yang, Jwing-Ming's Long-Fist Grandmaster.

**Hangzhou** (杭州). A Chinese city in Zhejiang Province (浙江省).

**He, Zhu** (何鑄). An officer who was assigned as an investigator for Marshal Yue, Fei's case during the Chinese Song dynasty (宋).

**Henan Province** (河南省). A province in China.

**hou tian qi** (後天氣). Post-birth qi. This qi is converted from the essence of food and air and is classified as "fire qi" (huo qi, 火氣) since it can make your body too yang.

**hu bu gong** (虎步功). Tiger step gong, a style of qigong training.

**Hua Tuo** (華陀). A well-known physician who lived during the Chinese Jin dynasty (晉) in the third century AD.

**huan jing bu nao** (還精補腦). "To return the essence to nourish the brain." A Daoist qigong training process wherein qi that is converted from essence is led to the brain to nourish it.

**huan** (緩). Slow.

**huiyin (Co-1)** (會陰). An acupuncture cavity belonging to the conception vessel (ren mai, 任脈).

**huo long gong** (火龍功). Fire dragon gong. A style of qigong training created by Taiyang martial stylists (太陽宗).

**huo lu** (火路). Called the fire path, one of the paths in Small Circulation (Xiao Zhou Tian, 小周天) Meditation.

**jian jue** (劍訣). Sword secret. A special hand posture in which the index and middle fingers are extended while the other three fingers touch each other.

**jiao hua gong** (叫化功). Beggar gong, a style of qigong training.

**Jin dynasty** (金). A dynasty in China, (AD 1115–1234).

**Jin dynasty** (晉). Chinese dynasty in the third century AD.

***Jin Kui Yao Lue*** (金匱要略). *Prescriptions from the Golden Chamber*, a book written by Zhang, Zhong-jing (張仲景) during the Chinese Qin and Han dynasties (秦，漢) (220 BC–AD 221). It discusses the use of breathing and acupuncture to maintain good qi flow. See also **Zhang, Zhong-jing**.

**jin pai** (金牌). Jin pai was the emperor's official seal that verified that the order was from the emperor himself.

**Jin, Shao-feng** (金紹峰). Dr. Yang, Jwing-Ming's White Crane grandmaster.

**jing** (精). Essence. The most refined part of anything.

**jing** (靜). Calm and silent.

**jing** (經). Called channels, but also translated as meridian. Refers to the twelve organ-related "rivers" which circulate qi throughout the body.

**jingmen** (精門). These are the essence doors, two cavities located in the kidney area at the back of the body.

**jing qi** (精氣). Essence qi, which has been converted from original essence.

**jing zi** (精子). The essence of the son," because it contains the jing of the father, which is passed on to his son (or daughter) and becomes the son's jing.

**ju jing hui shen** (聚精會神). Means gathering your jing to meet your shen, which implies concentration.

**Jun Qing** (君倩). A Daoist and Chinese doctor from the Chinese Jin dynasty (AD 265–420, 晉), who is credited with being the creator of the Five Animal Sports Qigong (Wu Qin Xi, 五禽戲) practice.

**Kao, Tao** (高濤). Dr. Yang, Jwing-Ming's first Taijiquan master.

**kung** (功). See **gong**.

**kung fu** (功夫). See **gongfu**.

**kuoshu** (國術). National techniques, another name for Chinese martial arts. First used by President Chiang, Kai-Shek (蔣介石) in 1926 at the founding of the Nanking Central Guoshu Institute (南京中央國術館). Also see **guoshu**.

***Lan Shi Mi Cang*** (蘭室祕藏). *Secret Library of the Orchid Room*. Chinese medical and qigong book written by Li, Guo (李果) that describes using qigong and herbal remedies for internal disorders. See also **Li, Guo**.

**Lao Zi (Li, Er)** (老子). The creator of scholarly Daoism; nickname was Li, Er (李耳).

**Li, Guo** (李果). Chinese physician and qigong master who wrote the book, *Secret Library of the Orchid Room* (*Lan Shi Mi Cang*, 蘭室祕藏) during the period of the Song, Jin, and Yuan dynasties (宋，金，元) (AD 960–1368). See also ***Lan Shi Mi Cang.***

**Li, Mao-Ching** (李茂清). Dr. Yang, Jwing-Ming's Long Fist master.

**Li, Qing-an** (李清菴). Qigong master from the Chinese Yuan dynasty (元).

**Liang dynasty** (梁). Chinese dynasty, (AD 502–557).

**luo** (絡). The small qi channels that branch out from the primary qi channels and are connected to the skin and to the bone marrow.

**mai** (脈). Means "vessel" or "qi channel."

**mian** (綿). Soft.

**Ming dynasty** (明朝). Chinese dynasty, (AD 1368–1644).

**ming tian gu** (鳴天鼓). To beat the heavenly drum, a qigong practice for waking up and clearing the mind in which the back of the head is tapped with the fingers.

**mingmen (Gv-4)** (命門). An acupuncture cavity belonging to the governing vessel (du mai, 督脈).

***Nan Jing*** (難經). *Classic on Disorders,* medical book written by Bian Que during the Qin and Han dynasties, which describes methods of using breathing to increase qi circulation. See also **Brian Que**.

**Nan Song** (南宋). "Southern Song." After the Song dynasty was conquered by the Jin race from Mongolia, the Song people moved south and established another country, called Southern Song, (AD 1127–1279).

**nei dan** (內丹). A form of qigong in which qi (the elixir) is built up in the body and spread out to the limbs.

***Nei Gong Tu Shuo*** (內功圖說). *Illustrated Explanation of Nei Gong.* A qigong book written by Wang, Zu-yuan (王祖源) during the Qing dynasty. This book presents the Twelve Pieces of Brocade and explains the idea of combining both moving and stationary qigong.

**nei shi gongfu** (內視功夫). Nei shi means to look internally, so nei shi gongfu refers to the art of looking inside yourself to read the state of your health and the condition of your qi.

**qi** (氣). Qi is universal energy, including heat, light, and electromagnetic energy. Qi also refers to the energy circulating in human and animal bodies. A current popular model is that the qi circulating in the human body is bioelectric in nature. Also called chi.

***Qi Hua Lun*** (氣化論). *Qi Variation Thesis.* An ancient treatise that discusses the variations of qi in the universe.

**qi huo** (起火). To start a fire is the analogy used in qigong practice when you start to build up qi at the lower dan tian (xia dan tian, 下丹田).

**qi lun** (臍輪). Called a "belly wheel," it is a term that the Daoists commonly use for the navel. The Daoists, like the Buddhists, believe that people die and are reborn repeatedly in cycles that move like a great wheel. The abdomen, specifically the navel area, is strongly involved in this reincarnation.

***Qian Jin Fang*** (千金方). *Thousand Gold Prescriptions.* A medical book that describes the method of leading qi, and also describes the use of the six sounds (liu sheng, 六聲). It was written by Sun, Si-miao (孫思邈), a physician during the Sui and Tang dynasties (隋，唐) (AD 581–907). Also see **Sun, Si-miao**.

**qigong** (氣功). Gong means gongfu (energy-time). Qigong means study, research, and/ or practices related to qi. Also called chi kung.

**qigong an mo** (氣功按摩). Qigong massage.

**qihai (Co-6)** (氣海). An acupuncture cavity belonging to the conception vessel (ren mai, 任脈).

**Qin dynasty** (秦朝). Chinese dynasty, (255–206 BC).

**Qin, Kuai** (秦檜). The prime minister of the Southern Song dynasty (南宋).

**qin na** (擒拿). See **chin na**.

**Qing dynasty** (清朝). Last Chinese dynasty, (AD 1644–1912).

**qing xiu pai** (清修派). The peaceful cultivation division of Daoist qigong training that is similar to that of Buddhism.

**ren** (人). Man or mankind.

**Ren (Chan)** (禪 or 忍) A Chinese school of Mahayana Buddhism, which asserts that enlightenment can be attained through meditation, self-contemplation, and intuition, rather than through study of scripture. Ren (Chan) is commonly known as Zen in Japan.

**ren mai** (任脈). Conception vessel, one of the eight extraordinary vessels.

**ren qi** (人氣). Human qi.

**ren shi** (人事). Human events, activities, and relationships.

**Ren Zong** (仁宗). Emperor of the Song dynasty (宋) (AD 1023–1064).

***Ru Men Shi Shi*** (儒門視事). *The Confucian Point of View*, a book written by Zhang, Zi-he advocated using qigong to cure external injuries; written during the Song, Jin, and Yuan dynasties (宋，金，元) (AD 960–1368). See also **Zhang, Zi-he**.

**san bao** (三寶). Three treasures: human essence (jing, 精), energy (qi, 氣) and spirit (shen, 神). Also called san yuan (three origins, 三元).

**san ben** (三本). The three foundations.

**san cai** (三才). Three powers, heaven, earth, and man.

**sanjiao** (三焦).The triple burner. In Chinese medicine, the body is divided into three sections: the upper burner (shang jiao, 上焦) (chest); the middle burner (zhong jiao, 中焦) (stomach area); and the lower burner (xia jiao, 下焦) (lower abdomen).

**shang dan tian** (上丹田). Upper dan tian. Located at the third eye, it is the residence of the spirit (shen, 神).

**Shang dynasty** (商朝). Chinese dynasty, (1766–1154 BC).

**Shaolin Temple** (少林寺). A monastery located in Henan Province (河南省), China that is well-known because of its martial arts training.

**shen** (神). Spirit. According to Chinese qigong, the shen resides at the upper dan tian (shang dan tian, 上丹田) and is called the third eye.

**shen** (深). Deep.

**shen xin ping heng** (身心平衡). Body and heart (mind) balanced, which means the balance of physical body and the mental body.

**shenshu (B-23)** (腎俞). An acupuncture cavity belonging to the bladder qi channel (膀胱經).

**shi er zhuang** (十二庄). Twelve Postures. A style of qigong practice created during the Chinese Qing dynasty (清).

*Shi Ji* (史紀). *Historical Record.* A book written in the Spring and Autumn and Warring States Periods (春秋戰國) (770–221 BC).

**shui lu** (水路). Water path. One of the meditation paths in which the qi is led upward through the spinal cord to nourish the brain.

**Song dynasty** (宋朝) Dynasty in Chinese history from (AD 960–1279).

**Southern Song dynasty** (南宋). After the Song dynasty was conquered by the Jin race from Mongolia, the Song people moved to the south and established another country, called Southern Song, from (AD 1127–1279).

**suan ming shi** (算命師). Calculate life teacher, a fortune teller who is able to calculate your future and destiny.

**Sui dynasty** (隋). A Chinese dynasty, (AD 581–618).

*Sun Zi Bing Fa* (孫子兵法). *Sun's Book of Tactics,* Military book written by Sun, Wu (孫武), c. 557 BC.

**Sun, Si-miao** (孫思邈). A well-known Chinese physician and qigong master who wrote the book, *Thousand Gold Prescriptions* (*Qian Jin Fang*, 千金方) during the Sui and Tang dynasties (AD 581–907).

**Sun, Wu** (孫武). Military strategist who wrote *Sun's Book of Tactics* (*Sun Zi Bing Fa*, 孫子兵法), c. 557 BC.

**tai chi chuan (taijiquan)** (太極拳). A Chinese internal martial style based on the theory of taiji (grand ultimate, 太極).

**taiji** (太極). Means "grand ultimate," the force which generates two poles, yin and yang.

**Taiyang martial stylists** (太陽宗). A school of Chinese martial arts that trains Fire Dragon Gong (火龍功).

**Taizuquan** (太祖拳). A style of Chinese external martial arts.

**Tang dynasty** (唐朝). A dynasty in Chinese history from (AD 618–907).

**Tang Yin Xian** (湯陰縣). A county in Henan Province that is Marshal Yue, Fei's birthplace.

**Tao, Hong-jing** (陶弘景) (AD 456–536). Physician and qigong master who compiled the book, *Records of Nourishing the Body and Extending Life* (*Yang Shen Yan Ming Lu*, 養身延命錄).

**Teng Pai Jun** (籐牌軍). The Rattan Shield Army, a special fighting unit trained by Marshal Yue, Fei (岳飛) to fight against guai zi ma (枴子馬).

**teng** (籐). Rattan.

**tian** (天). Heaven or sky.

**tian ling gai** (天靈蓋). Called "heaven spiritual cover," it means crown of the head.

**tian qi** (天氣). Heaven qi. It is now commonly used to mean the weather, since weather is governed by heaven qi.

**tian shi** (天時). Heavenly timing. The repeating natural cycles generated by the heavens, such as seasons, months, days, and hours.

**tian zhu** (天柱). Refers to "heaven pillar," which means the two muscles on the back of the neck that support the head (i.e., heaven).

**tiao qi** (調氣). To regulate the qi.

**tiao shen** (調身). To regulate the body.

**tiao shen** (調神). To regulate the spirit.

**tiao xi** (調息). To regulate the breathing.

**tiao xin** (調心). To regulate the emotional mind.

**tie bu shan** (鐵布衫). Gongfu training that toughens the body externally and internally is called "iron shirt".

***Tong Ren Yu Xue Zhen Jiu Tu*** (銅人俞穴鍼灸圖). *Illustration of the Brass Man Acupuncture and Moxibustion,* an acupuncture book written by Dr. Wang, Wei-yi (王唯一) during the Song dynasty. See also **Wang, Wei-yi.**

**tui na** (推拿). Means "to push and grab," a category of Chinese massage for treating injuries and promoting healing.

**wai dan** (外丹). External (elixir) qigong exercises in which a practitioner will build up the qi in his limbs and then lead it into the center of his body for nourishment.

***Wai Tai Mi Yao*** (外台祕要). *The Extra Important Secret.* A Chinese medical book written by Wang, Tao (王燾), this book discusses the use of breathing and herbal therapies for qi circulation disorders. See also **Wang, Tao.**

**Wang, Tao** (王燾).Chinese physician and qigong master who wrote the book *The Extra Important Secret* (*Wai Tai Mi Yao,* 外台祕要) during the Sui and Tang dynasties (隋，唐) (AD 581–907).

**Wang, Fan-an** (汪汎庵). Chinese physician who wrote the book *The Total Introduction to Medical Prescriptions* (*Yi Fan Ji Jie,* 醫方集介) during the Qing dynasty.

**Wang, Wei-yi** (王唯一). Chinese physician who wrote the book, *Illustration of the Brass Man Acupuncture and Moxibustion* (*Tong Ren Yu Xue Zhen Jiu Tu,* 銅人俞穴鍼灸圖) and systematically organized acupuncture theory and principles.

**Wang, Zu-yuan** (王祖源). Chinese physician who wrote the book, *Illustrated Explanation of Nei Gong* (*Nei Gong Tu Shuo,* 內功圖說) during the Qing dynasty (清).

**wei qi** (衛氣). Protective qi or guardian qi. The qi at the surface of the body that generates a shield to protect the body from negative external influences, such as colds.

**Wei, Bo-yang** (魏伯陽). A physician who wrote the book, *A Comparative Study of the Zhou (dynasty) Book of Changes* (*Zhou Yi Can Tong Qi,* 周易參同契) during the Qin and Han dynasties (秦，漢) (221 BC–AD 220).

**Wu Qin Xi** (五禽戲). Five Animal Sports, a medical qigong practice created by Jun Qing (君倩) during the Chinese Jin dynasty, (晉) (AD 265–420)

**Wu Zhen Ren** (伍真人). The Daoist name of Wu, Shou-yang (AD 1552–1640), a well-known Daoist qigong master from the Chinese Ming dynasty (明).

**Wu Zhu** (兀朮). A general of the Jin (金) at the time of the Chinese Southern Song dynasty (南宋).

**wushu** (武術). A common name for the Chinese martial arts. Many other terms are used, including (wuyi, 武藝), for martial arts; (wugong, 武功) for martial gongfu; (guoshu, 國術), for national techniques; and (gongfu, 功夫), which refers to energy-time. Because wushu has been modified into gymnastic martial performance in mainland China over the past forty years, many traditional Chinese martial artists have given up the name "wushu" to avoid confusing modern wushu with traditional wushu. Recently, mainland China has attempted to return modern wushu to its traditional training and practice.

**xi** (細). Slender.

**Xi Sui Jing** (洗髓經). *Washing Marrow/Brain Classic*, usually translated "*Marrow/Brain Washing Classic.*" A qigong training that specializes in leading qi to the marrow to cleanse it or to the brain to nourish the spirit for enlightenment. It is believed that Xi Sui Jing training is the key to longevity and achieving spiritual enlightenment.

**xia dan tian** (下丹). Lower dan tian. Located in the lower abdomen, the lower dan tian is believed to be the residence of water qi, original qi, (yuan qi, 元氣).

**xia jiao** (下焦). Lower burner. The lower abdomen is called the lower burner.

**xian tian qi** (先天氣). Pre-birth qi or pre-heaven qi, also called dan tian qi. It is the qi that is converted from original essence and is stored in the lower dan tian. Considered to be water qi, it is able to calm the body.

**xiao zhou tian** (小周天). Called small heavenly cycle, also called "small circulation." In qigong, when you can use your mind to lead qi through the conception and governing vessels, (任, 督脈) you have completed the cycle.

**Xiao Zong** (孝宗). Emperor of the Southern Song dynasty (南宋) (AD 1163–1190).

**xin huo** (心火). Heart fire.

**xin xi xiang yi** (心息相依). The heart (mind) and breathing (are) mutually dependent.

**Xingyiquan (hsing yi chuan)** (形意拳). Means "shape-mind fist," an internal style of gongfu in which the mind or thinking determines the shape or movement of the body. Creation of the style is attributed to Marshal Yue, Fei (岳飛).

**Xinzhu Xian** (新竹縣). Birthplace of Dr. Yang, Jwing-Ming in Taiwan.

**yang** (陽). In Chinese philosophy, this is the active, positive, masculine polarity. In Chinese medicine, yang means excessive, overactive, overheated. The yang (or outer) organs are the gall bladder, small intestine, large intestine, stomach, bladder, and triple burner.

*Yang Sheng Fu Yu* (養生膚語). *Brief Introduction to Nourishing the Body,* book by Chen, Ji-ru (陳繼儒) during the Qing dynasty (清). See also **Chen, Ji-ru.**

*Yang Shen Jue* (養生訣). *Life Nourishing Secrets,* medical book by Zhang, An Dao that discusses several qigong practices.written during the Song, Jin, and Yuan dynasties (宋，金，元) (AD 960–1368). See also **Zhang, An-dao.**

*Yang Shen Yan Ming Lu* (養身延命錄). *Records of Nourishing the Body and Extending Life.* A Chinese medical book written by Tao, Hong-jing (陶弘景) during the period (AD 420–581).

**Yang, Jwing-Ming** (楊俊敏). Author of this book.

**yi** (意). The mind that is generated by clear thinking and judgment, and which is able to make you calm, peaceful, and wise.

*Yi Fang Ji Jie* (醫方集介). *The Total Introduction to Medical Prescriptions,* Chinese medical book written by Wang, Fan-an (汪汎庵) during the Qing dynasty (清).

*Yi Jin Jing* (易筋經). *The Changing Muscle/Tendon Classic,* credited to Da Mo, written around AD 550, this work discusses wai dan qigong training for strengthening the physical body.

*Yi Jing* (易經). *Book of Changes,* book of divination written during the Zhou dynasty (周) (1122–934 BC).

**yi shou dan tian** (意守丹田). Keep your yi on your lower dan tian. In qigong training, you keep your mind at the lower dan tian in order to build up qi. When you are circulating your qi, you always lead your qi back to your lower dan tian (xia dan tian, 下丹田) before you stop.

**yi yi yin qi** (以意引氣). Use your yi (wisdom mind) to lead your qi, a qigong technique. Yi cannot be pushed, but it can be led. This is best done with the yi.

**Yin** (陰). In Chinese philosophy, this is the passive, negative, feminine polarity. In Chinese medicine, yin means deficient. The yin (internal) organs are the heart, lungs, liver, kidneys, spleen, and pericardium.

**ying qi** (營氣). This is the qi which manages the functioning of the organs and the body.

**yongquan (K-1)** (湧泉). Called the bubbling well, it is an acupuncture cavity belonging to the kidney primary qi channel.

**you** (悠). Long, far, meditative, continuous, slow and soft.

**Yuan dynasty** (元代). A Chinese dynasty AD 1206–1367.

**yuan jing** (元精). This is original essence, the fundamental, original substance inherited from your parents that is converted into original qi.

**yuan qi** (元氣). This is original qi, which is created from the original essence inherited from your parents.

**Yue, Fei** (岳飛). A Chinese hero from the Southern Song dynasty (南宋) (AD 1127–1279). He is said to have created Ba Duan Jin (八段錦), Xingyiquan (形意拳), and Yue's Ying Zhua (岳家鷹爪).

**Yue Jia Jun** (岳家軍). Name given to Marshal Yue, Fei's troops.

**Yue Wu Mu** (岳武穆). Means "Yue, the righteous and respectable warrior." An honorable title given to Marshal Yue, Fei by the Southern Song emperor Xiao Zong (孝宗).

**Yue, Yun** (岳雲). Yue, Fei's adopted son. He was also killed when Yue, Fei was murdered.

**yun** (勻). Uniform or even.

**Zen** (忍). To endure. The Japanese name of Chan (禪). See also **Chan**.

**Zhang, An-dao** (張安道). Chinese physician and qigong master who wrote *Life Nourishing Secrets* (*Yang Shen Jue,* 養生訣), during the Song, Jin, and Yuan dynasties. See also *Yang Shen Jue.*

**Zhang, Dao-ling** (張道陵). Combined scholarly Daoism with Buddhist philosophies, created Religious Daoism (Dao Jiao, 道教) sometime during the Chinese Eastern Han dynasty (東漢) (AD 25–221).

**Zhang, San-feng** (張三豐). A Daoist qigong and martial arts master who was credited as the creator of taijiquan (太極拳) during the Chinese Song dynasty (宋).

**Zhang,, Xian** (張憲). Yue, Fei's top military officer. He was also killed when Yue, Fei was murdered.

**Zhang, Zhong-jing** (張仲景). Chinese physician who wrote *Prescriptions from the Golden Chamber* (*Jin Kui Yao Lue*, 金匱要略), during the Qin and Han dynasties (秦，漢) (221 BC–AD 220,).

**Zhang, Zi-he** (張子和). Chinese physician (AD 1156–1228) who wrote *The Confucian Point of View* (*Ru Men Shi Shi*, 儒門視事), which advocates the use of qigong to cure external injuries such as cuts and sprains. See also *Ru Men Shi Shi.*

**zhong dan tian** (中丹田). Middle dan tian that is located in the area of the solar plexus; it is the residence of fire qi.

**zhong jiao** (中焦). Middle burner (*sanjiao*), one of the triple burners.

**Zhou dynasty** (周朝). A dynasty in China, (1122–934 BC).

**Zhou, Tong** (周侗). Marshal Yue, Fei's martial arts teacher.

***Zhou Yi Can Tong Qi* (**周易參同契). *A Comparative Study of the Zhou (dynasty) Book of Changes*, a medical and qigong book written by Wei, Bo-yang that discusses the relationship of human beings to nature's forces and qi. See also **Wei, Bo-yang**.

***Zhu Bing Yuan Hou Lun*** (諸病源候論). Book of 260 different ways of increasing the qi flow. See also **Chao, Yuan-fang**.

**Zhu, Dan-xi** (朱丹溪). Chinese physician who wrote *A Further Thesis of Complete Study*, during Chinese Song, Jin, and Yuan dynasties (宋，金，元) (AD 960–1368). See also *Ge Zhi Yu Lun.*

**Zhuang Zhou** (莊周). Contemporary of Mencius who advocated Daoism.

# Index

# About the Author

## Yang, Jwing-Ming, PhD (楊俊敏博士)

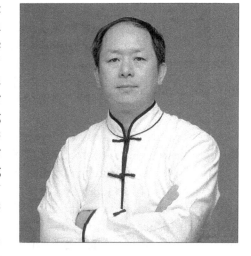

Dr. Yang, Jwing-Ming was born on August 11, 1946, in Xinzhu Xian (新竹縣), Taiwan (台灣), Republic of China (中華民國). He started his wushu (武術) (*gongfu* or *kung fu*, 功夫) training at the age of fifteen under Shaolin White Crane (*Bai He*, 少林白鶴) Master Cheng, Gin-Gsao (曾金灶). Master Cheng originally learned Taizuquan (太祖拳) from his grandfather when he was a child. When Master Cheng was fifteen years old, he started learning White Crane from Master Jin, Shao-Feng (金紹峰), and followed him for twenty-three years until Master Jin's death.

In thirteen years of study (1961–1974) under Master Cheng, Dr. Yang became an expert in the White Crane style of Chinese martial arts, which includes both the use of bare hand and various weapons, such as saber, staff, spear, trident, two short rods, and many other weapons. With the same master he also studied White Crane Qigong (氣功), *qin na* or *chin na* (擒拿), *tui na* (推拿), and *dian xue* massages (點穴按摩), and herbal treatment.

At the age of sixteen, Dr. Yang began the study of Yang Style Taijiquan (楊氏太極拳) under Master Kao, Tao (高濤). After learning from Master Kao, Dr. Yang continued his study and research of taijiquan with several masters and senior practitioners such as Master Li, Mao-Ching (李茂清) and Mr. Wilson Chen (陳威伸) in Taipei (台北). Master Li learned his taijiquan from the well-known Master Han, Ching-Tang (韓慶堂), and Mr. Chen learned his taijiquan from Master Chang, Xiang-San (張詳三). Dr. Yang has mastered the taiji bare hand sequence, pushing hands, the two-man fighting sequence, taiji sword, taiji saber, and taiji qigong.

When Dr. Yang was eighteen years old, he entered Tamkang College (淡江學院) in Taipei Xian to study physics. In college he began the study of traditional Shaolin Long Fist (*Changquan* or *Chang Chuan*, 少林長拳) with Master Li, Mao-Ching at the Tamkang College Guoshu Club (淡江國術社), 1964–1968, and eventually became an assistant instructor under Master Li. In 1971, he completed his MS degree in physics at the National Taiwan University (台灣大學) and then served in the Chinese Air Force from 1971 to 1972. In the service, Dr. Yang taught physics at the Junior Academy of the Chinese Air Force (空軍幼校) while also teaching wushu. After being honorably discharged in 1972, he returned to Tamkang College to teach physics and resumed study under Master Li, Mao-Ching. From Master Li, Dr. Yang learned northern style wushu, which includes both bare hand and kicking techniques, and numerous weapons.

In 1974, Dr. Yang came to the United States to study mechanical engineering at Purdue University. At the request of a few students, Dr. Yang began to teach gongfu (*kung fu*), which resulted in the establishment of the Purdue University Chinese Kung Fu Research Club in the spring of 1975. While at Purdue, Dr. Yang also taught college-credit courses in taijiquan. In May of 1978, he was awarded a PhD in mechanical engineering from Purdue.

In 1980, Dr. Yang moved to Houston to work for Texas Instruments. While in Houston, he founded Yang's Shaolin Kung Fu Academy, which was eventually taken over by his disciple Mr. Jeffery Bolt after Dr. Yang moved to Boston in 1982. Dr. Yang founded Yang's Martial Arts Academy in Boston on October 1, 1982.

In January of 1984, he gave up his engineering career to devote more time to research, writing, and teaching. In March of 1986, he purchased property in the Jamaica Plain area of Boston to be used as the headquarters of the new organization, Yang's Martial Arts Association (YMAA). The organization expanded to become a division of Yang's Oriental Arts Association, Inc. (YOAA).

In 2004, Dr. Yang began the nonprofit YMAA California Retreat Center. This training facility in rural California is where selected students enroll in a 10-year residency to learn Chinese martial arts.

In summary, Dr. Yang has been involved in Chinese martial arts since 1961. During this time, he spent thirteen years learning Shaolin White Crane (*Bai He*), Shaolin Long Fist (*Changquan*), and taijiquan. Dr. Yang has more than four decades of teaching experience.

In addition, Dr. Yang has also offered seminars around the world to share his knowledge of Chinese martial arts and qigong. The countries he has visited include Canada, Mexico, France, Italy, Poland, England, Ireland, Portugal, Switzerland, Germany, Hungary, Spain, Holland, Latvia, South Africa, and Saudi Arabia.

Since 1986, YMAA has become an international organization, which currently includes more than fifty schools located in Argentina, Belgium, Canada, Chile, France, Hungary, Iran, Ireland, Italy, New Zealand, Poland, Portugal, South Africa, Sweden, United Kingdom, Venezuela, and the United States. Many of Dr. Yang's books and videotapes have been translated into languages such as French, Italian, Spanish, Polish, Czech, Bulgarian, Russian, German, and Hungarian.

**Books written by Dr. Yang, Jwing-Ming**

1. *Shaolin Chin Na*, Unique Publications, Inc., 1980

2. *Shaolin Long Fist Kung Fu*, Unique Publications, Inc., 1981

3. *Yang Style Tai Chi Chuan*, Unique Publications, Inc., 1981

4. *Introduction to Ancient Chinese Weapons*, Unique Publications, Inc., 1985

5. *A Martial Arists Guide to Ancient Chinese Weapons*, revised edition, YMAA Publication Center, 1999

6. *Chi Kung for Health and Martial Arts*, YMAA Publication Center, 1985

7. *Qigong—Health and Martial Arts*, revised edition, YMAA Publication Center, 1998

8. *Northern Shaolin Sword*, YMAA Publication Center, 1985

9. *Advanced Yang Style Tai Chi Chuan Vol. 1—Tai Chi Theory and Martial Power*, YMAA Publication Center, 1986

10. *Tai Chi Theory and Martial Power*, revised edition, YMAA Publication Center, 1996

11. *Advanced Yang Style Tai Chi Chuan Vol. 2—Tai Chi Chuan Martial Applications*, YMAA Publication Center, 1986

12. *Tai Chi Chuan Martial Applications*, revised edition, YMAA Publication Center, 1996

13. *Analysis of Shaolin Chin Na*, YMAA Publication Center, 1987, 2004

14. *The Eight Pieces of Brocade—Ba Duan Jin*, YMAA Publication Center, 1988

15. *Eight Simple Qigong Exercises for Health*, revised edition, YMAA Publication Center, 1997

16. *The Root of Chinese Qigong—The Secrets of Qigong Training*, YMAA Publication Center, 1989, 1997

17. *Muscle/Tendon Changing and Marrow/Brain Washing Chi Kung—The Secret of Youth*, YMAA Publication Center, 1989

18. *Qigong the Secret of Youth, Da Mo's Muscle Tendon Changing and Marrow Brain Washing Qigong*, revised edition, YMAA Publication Center, 2000

19. *Hsing Yi Chuan—Theory and Applications*, YMAA Publication Center, 1990

20. *Xingyiquan—Theory and Applications*, revised edition, YMAA Publication Center, 2003

21. *The Essence of Tai Chi Chi Kung—Health and Martial Arts*, YMAA Publication Center, 1990

22. *The Essence of Taiji Qigong—Health and Martial Arts*, revised edition, YMAA Publication Center, 1998

23. *Qigong for Arthritis*, YMAA Publication Center, 1991

24. *Arthritis Relief,* revised edition, YMAA Publication Center, 2005

25. *Chinese Qigong Massage—General Massage,* YMAA Publication Center, 1992

26. *Qigong Massage—Fundamental Techniques for Health and Relaxation,* revised edition, YMAA Publication Center, 2005

27. *How to Defend Yourself,* YMAA Publication Center, 1992

28. *Baguazhang—Emei Baguazhang,* YMAA Publication Center, 1994

29. *Baguazhang—Theory and Applications,* revised edition, YMAA Publication Center, 2008

30. *Comprehensive Applications of Shaolin Chin Na—The Practical Defense of Chinese Seizing Arts,* YMAA Publication Center, 1995

31. *Taiji Chin Na—The Seizing Art of Taijiquan,* YMAA Publication Center, 1995

32. *The Essence of Shaolin White Crane,* YMAA Publication Center, 1996

33. *Back Pain—Chinese Qigong for Healing and Prevention,* YMAA Publication Center, 1997

34. *Back Pain Relief—Chinese Qigong for Healing and Prevention,* revised edition, YMAA Publication Center, 2004

35. *Taijiquan Classical Yang Style—The Complete Form and Qigong,* YMAA Publication Center, 1999

36. *Tai Chi Chuan—Classical Yang Style,* revised edition, YMAA Publication Center, 2010

37. *Taijiquan Theory of Dr. Yang, Jwing-Ming—The Root of Taijiquan,* YMAA Publication Center, 2003

38. *Qigong Meditation—Embryonic Breathing,* YMAA Publication Center, 2003

39. *Qigong Meditation—Small Circulation,* YMAA Publication Center, 2006

40. *Tai Chi Ball Qigong—Health and Martial Arts,* YMAA Publication Center, 2010

## DVD Videos by Dr. Yang, Jwing-Ming

1. *Chin Na In Depth Courses 1–4,* YMAA Publication Center, 2003

2. *Chin Na In Depth Courses 5–8,* YMAA Publication Center, 2003

3. *Chin Na In Depth Courses 9–12,* YMAA Publication Center, 2003

4. *Eight Simple Qigong Exercises for Health—The Eight Pieces of Brocade,* YMAA Publication Center, 2003

5. *Shaolin White Crane Gong Fu Basic Training Courses 1 & 2,* YMAA Publication Center, 2003

6. *Shaolin White Crane Hard and Soft Qigong,* YMAA Publication Center, 2003

7. *Tai Chi Chuan Classical Yang Style* (long form Taijiquan), YMAA Publication Center, 2003

8. *Analysis of Shaolin Chin Na,* YMAA Publication Center, 2004

9. *Shaolin Kung Fu Fundamental Training,* YMAA Publication Center, 2004

10. *Baguazhang (8 Trigrams Palm Kung Fu),* YMAA Publication Center, 2005

11. *Essence of Taiji Qigong,* YMAA Publication Center, 2005

12. *Qigong Massage,* YMAA Publication Center, 2005

13. *Shaolin Long Fist Kung Fu Basic Sequences,* YMAA Publication Center, 2005

14. *Taiji Pushing Hands Courses 1 & 2,* YMAA Publication Center, 2005

15. *Taiji Sword, Classical Yang Style,* YMAA Publication Center, 2005

16. *Taiji Ball Qigong Courses 1 & 2,* YMAA Publication Center, 2006

17. *Taiji Fighting Set—88 Posture,* 2–Person Matching Set, YMAA Publication Center, 2006

18. *Taiji Pushing Hands Courses 3 & 4,* YMAA Publication Center, 2006

19. *Understanding Qigong DVD 1—What is Qigong? Understanding the Human Qi Circulatory System,* YMAA Publication Center, 2006

20. *Understanding Qigong DVD 2—Keypoints of Qigong & Qigong Breathing,* YMAA Publication Center, 2006

21. *Shaolin Saber Basic Sequences,* YMAA Publication Center, 2007

22. *Shaolin Staff Basic Sequences,* YMAA Publication Center, 2007

23. *Simple Qigong Exercises for Arthritis Relief,* YMAA Publication Center, 2007

24. *Simple Qigong Exercises for Back Pain Relief,* YMAA Publication Center, 2007

25. *Taiji & Shaolin Staff Fundamental Training,* YMAA Publication Center, 2007

26. *Taiji Ball Qigong Courses 3 & 4,* YMAA Publication Center, 2007

27. *Understanding Qigong DVD 3—Embryonic Breathing,* YMAA Publication Center, 2007

28. *Understanding Qigong DVD 4—Four Seasons Qigong,* YMAA Publication Center, 2007

29. *Understanding Qigong DVD 5—Small Circulation,* YMAA Publication Center, 2007

30. *Understanding Qigong DVD 6—Martial Arts Qigong Breathing,* YMAA Publication Center, 2007

31. *Five Animal Sports Qigong,* YMAA Publication Center, 2008

32. *Saber Fundamental Training,* YMAA Publication Center, 2008

33. *Shaolin White Crane Gong Fu Basic Training Courses 3 & 4,* YMAA Publication Center, 2008

34. *Taiji 37 Postures Martial Applications,* YMAA Publication Center, 2008

35. *Taiji Saber, Classical Yang Style,* YMAA Publication Center, 2008

36. *Taiji Wrestling— Advanced Takedown Techniques,* YMAA Publication Center, 2008

37. *Taiji Yin/Yang Sticking Hands,* YMAA Publication Center, 2008

38. *Xingyiquan (Hsing I Chuan),* YMAA Publication Center, 2008

39. *Northern Shaolin Sword,* YMAA Publication Center, 2009

40. *Sword Fundamental Training,* YMAA Publication Center, 2009

41. *Taiji Chin Na in Depth,* YMAA Publication Center, 2009

42. *YMAA 25-Year Anniversary,* YMAA Publication Center, 2009

43. *Shuai Jiao–Kung Fu Wrestling,* YMAA Publication Center, 2010

44. *Knife Defense—Traditional Techniques,* YMAA Publication Center, 2011

45. *Yang Tai Chi for Beginners,* YMAA Publication Center, 2012

6 HEALING MOVEMENTS

101 REFLECTIONS ON TAI CHI CHUAN

108 INSIGHTS INTO TAI CHI CHUAN

ADVANCING IN TAE KWON DO

ANALYSIS OF SHAOLIN CHIN NA 2ND ED

ANCIENT CHINESE WEAPONS

ART OF HOJO UNDO

ARTHRITIS RELIEF, 3RD ED.

BACK PAIN RELIEF, 2ND ED.

BAGUAZHANG, 2ND ED.

CARDIO KICKBOXING ELITE

CHIN NA IN GROUND FIGHTING

CHINESE FAST WRESTLING

CHINESE FITNESS

CHINESE TUI NA MASSAGE

CHOJUN

COMPREHENSIVE APPLICATIONS OF SHAOLIN
    CHIN NA

CONFLICT COMMUNICATION

CROCODILE AND THE CRANE: A NOVEL

CUTTING SEASON: A XENON PEARL MARTIAL
    ARTS THRILLER

DESHI: A CONNOR BURKE MARTIAL ARTS THRILLER

DIRTY GROUND

DR. WU'S HEAD MASSAGE

DUKKHA REVERB

DUKKHA, THE SUFFERING: AN EYE FOR AN EYE

DUKKHA UNLOADED

ENZAN: THE FAR MOUNTAIN, A CONNOR BURKE MARTIAL ARTS THRILLER

ESSENCE OF SHAOLIN WHITE CRANE

EXPLORING TAI CHI

FACING VIOLENCE

FIGHT LIKE A PHYSICIST

FIGHTING ARTS

FIRST DEFENSE

FORCE DECISIONS: A CITIZENS GUIDE

FOX BORROWS THE TIGER'S AWE

INSIDE TAI CHI

KAGE: THE SHADOW, A CONNOR BURKE MARTIAL ARTS THRILLER

KATA AND THE TRANSMISSION OF KNOWLEDGE

KRAV MAGA: WEAPON DEFENSES

LITTLE BLACK BOOK OF VIOLENCE

LIUHEBAFA FIVE CHARACTER SECRETS

MARTIAL ARTS ATHLETE

MARTIAL ARTS INSTRUCTION

MARTIAL WAY AND ITS VIRTUES

MASK OF THE KING

MEDITATIONS ON VIOLENCE

MIND/BODY FITNESS

THE MIND INSIDE TAI CHI

MUGAI RYU

NATURAL HEALING WITH QIGONG

NORTHERN SHAOLIN SWORD, 2ND ED.

OKINAWA'S COMPLETE KARATE SYSTEM: ISSHIN RYU

POWER BODY

PRINCIPLES OF TRADITIONAL CHINESE MEDICINE

QIGONG FOR HEALTH & MARTIAL ARTS 2ND ED.

QIGONG FOR LIVING

QIGONG FOR TREATING COMMON AILMENTS

QIGONG MASSAGE

QIGONG MEDITATION: EMBRYONIC BREATHING

QIGONG MEDITATION: SMALL CIRCULATION

QIGONG, THE SECRET OF YOUTH: DA MO'S CLASSICS

QUIET TEACHER: A XENON PEARL MARTIAL ARTS THRILLER

RAVEN'S WARRIOR

ROOT OF CHINESE QIGONG, 2ND ED.

SCALING FORCE

SENSEI: A CONNOR BURKE MARTIAL ARTS THRILLER

SHIHAN TE: THE BUNKAI OF KATA

SHIN GI TAI: KARATE TRAINING FOR BODY, MIND, AND SPIRIT

SIMPLE CHINESE MEDICINE

SIMPLE QIGONG EXERCISES FOR HEALTH, 3RD ED.

SIMPLIFIED TAI CHI CHUAN, 2ND ED.

SUDDEN DAWN: THE EPIC JOURNEY OF BODHIDHARMA

SUNRISE TAI CHI

SUNSET TAI CHI

SURVIVING ARMED ASSAULTS

TAE KWON DO: THE KOREAN MARTIAL ART

TAEKWONDO BLACK BELT POOMSAE

TAEKWONDO: A PATH TO EXCELLENCE

TAEKWONDO: ANCIENT WISDOM FOR THE MODERN WARRIOR

TAEKWONDO: DEFENSES AGAINST WEAPONS

TAEKWONDO: SPIRIT AND PRACTICE

TAO OF BIOENERGETICS

TAI CHI BALL QIGONG: FOR HEALTH AND MARTIAL ARTS

TAI CHI BOOK

TAI CHI CHIN NA: THE SEIZING ART OF TAI CHI CHUAN, 2ND ED.

TAI CHI CHUAN CLASSICAL YANG STYLE, 2ND ED.

TAI CHI CHUAN MARTIAL APPLICATIONS

TAI CHI CHUAN MARTIAL POWER, 3RD ED.

TAI CHI CONNECTIONS

TAI CHI DYNAMICS

TAI CHI QIGONG, 3RD ED.

TAI CHI SECRETS OF THE ANCIENT MASTERS

TAI CHI SECRETS OF THE WU & LI STYLES

TAI CHI SECRETS OF THE WU STYLE

TAI CHI SECRETS OF THE YANG STYLE

TAI CHI SWORD: CLASSICAL YANG STYLE, 2ND ED.

TAI CHI WALKING

TAIJIQUAN THEORY OF DR. YANG, JWING-MING

TENGU: THE MOUNTAIN GOBLIN, A CONNOR BURKE
    MARTIAL ARTS THRILLER

TRADITIONAL CHINESE HEALTH SECRETS

TRADITIONAL TAEKWONDO

WAY OF KATA

WAY OF KENDO AND KENJITSU

WAY OF SANCHIN KATA

WAY TO BLACK BELT

WESTERN HERBS FOR MARTIAL ARTISTS

WILD GOOSE QIGONG

WOMAN'S QIGONG GUIDE

XINGYIQUAN

continued on next page . . .

## DVDS FROM YMAA

more products available from . . .

**YMAA Publication Center, Inc.** 楊氏東方文化出版中心

1-800-669-8892 • info@ymaa.com • www.ymaa.com